W0234766

Nervous Disorders of Men

Born in Vienna in 1864, Bernard Hollander was a London-based psychiatrist in the early twentieth century. He is best known for being one of the main proponents of the interest in phrenology at that time. This title, originally published in 1916, looks at 'the numerous nervous illnesses of men, in which the *mental* factor plays a large part, and which are known as functional disorders, to distinguish them from organic diseases'. He looks at the role of psychotherapy as an emerging treatment for these disorders. There is also a companion volume which looks at the *Nervous Disorders of Women*.

Nervous Disorders of Men

The modern psychological conception of their causes, effects and rational treatment

Bernard Hollander

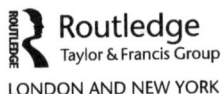

Routledge
Taylor & Francis Group

LONDON AND NEW YORK

First published in 1916
by Kegan Paul, Trench, Trubner & Co. Ltd

This edition first published in 2015 by Routledge
27 Church Road, Hove BN3 2FA

and by Routledge
711 Third Avenue, New York, NY 10017

Routledge is an imprint of the Taylor & Francis Group, an informa business

© 1916 Bernard Hollander

Publisher's Note
The publisher has gone to great lengths to ensure the quality of this
reprint but points out that some imperfections in the original copies may
be apparent.

Disclaimer
The publisher has made every effort to trace copyright holders and
welcomes correspondence from those they have been unable to contact.

ISBN: 978-1-138-80706-8 (hbk)
ISBN: 978-1-315-75125-2 (ebk)

NERVOUS
DISORDERS OF MEN

THE MODERN PSYCHOLOGICAL CONCEPTION
OF THEIR CAUSES, EFFECTS, AND
RATIONAL TREATMENT

BY

BERNARD HOLLANDER, M.D.

AUTHOR OF "THE MENTAL FUNCTIONS OF THE BRAIN",
"MENTAL SYMPTOMS OF BRAIN DISEASE",
"FIRST SIGNS OF INSANITY",
"HYPNOTISM AND SUGGESTION", ETC.

SECOND EDITION

LONDON
KEGAN PAUL, TRENCH, TRÜBNER & CO., LTD.
NEW YORK: E. P. DUTTON AND CO.
1916

BY THE SAME AUTHOR

NERVOUS DISORDERS OF WOMEN

THE MODERN PSYCHOLOGICAL CONCEPTION
OF THEIR CAUSES, EFFECTS, AND
RATIONAL TREATMENT.

ABNORMAL CHILDREN

(NERVOUS, MISCHIEVOUS, PRECOCIOUS, AND BACKWARD)

*A Book for Parents, Teachers,
and Medical Officers of Schools.*

ILLUSTRATED

First Edition   . February, 1916
Second Edition .   May, 1916

Printed in Great Britain

PREFACE

THIS book treats of the numerous nervous illnesses of men, in which the *mental* factor plays a large part, and which are known as functional disorders, to distinguish them from organic diseases. Until recently patients suffering from these disorders were not taken seriously, and their treatment is still left largely to men outside the profession. These are the patients who are attracted by patent medicine advertisements and by the numerous lay practitioners specialising in one form of treatment : in electricity, massage, physical exercise, diet treatment, or other specific ; or who have faith in "Christian Science," "Higher Thought," and other cults, and seek the treatment of "mental healers."

Now, however, that research into the functional disorders of the nervous system is carried on with the same zeal as into the organic disorders by physicians, eminent also as psychologists, and medical men are paying more and more attention to psychotherapy, there can be no longer any excuse for people exposing themselves to the dangers of treatment by unqualified persons. On the other hand, functional disorders occurring more in private than in hospital practice, and there being no systematic instruction in psychotherapy except in one or two of our Institutions, it is not only the lay public that has vague notions of this subject, but there must be also a large number of medical practitioners who lack the experience of its practical application and would like to learn what can be done by this mode of treatment for the benefit of the nervous sufferer. To them I address this book, not as a textbook, but rather as a series of essays on the various disorders of the nervous system, giving my personal observations and reflections, the result of long experience, and dwelling more especially on the *mental* causes and effects, and the counsels and treatment which I have found the most successful.

The book, being written in non-technical language and containing wholesome advice, should appeal also to those who have the care of nerve patients, and to other lay readers desirous of practical and useful information on the subject of nervous disorders. I am aware, of course, that every health teacher is confronted with the danger that his hygienic enlightenment may be sought by patients who are already dwelling too much on their troubles; but even these, I hope, may read the book with advantage, learning how nervous disorders may be caused and aggravated by unhealthy mental habits and profiting by the directions given for the acquisition of self-control.

This volume is limited to the discussion of nervous disorders peculiar to men, and is a companion volume to one on *Nervous Disorders of Women.* Of course, many of the complaints are common to both men and women, but their causation and to some extent their treatment is different in the two sexes and justifies the description being given in separate volumes.

BERNARD HOLLANDER, M.D.

57, WIMPOLE STREET,
LONDON, W.,
November, 1915.

CONTENTS

NERVOUS
DISORDERS OF MEN

CHAPTER I

"NERVOUSNESS," THE TENDENCY OF OUR AGE

IT is an often-repeated commonplace to-day,
that in consequence of the progress of civilisation
and the increase of brain activity entailed
thereby, nervousness in all its forms has become
much more common than formerly. We have
no statistics to prove the increase in the minor
nervous disorders; but as regards the severer
ones, such as the brain troubles resulting in
insanity, we have official figures at our disposal
which are distinctly startling. In 1860, for
instance, the proportion of insane to the normal
population was 1 in 536; in 1870 1 in 427; in
1880 1 in 357; in 1890 1 in 337; in 1900 1 in
289 and in 1910 it was 1 in 274, and in 1913 it
was 1 in 266. If the unofficial and borderland
cases were included, the ratio would be still more

B

alarming. But it is not insanity that we intend
to discuss, but the minor nervous disorders,
so-called functional disorders, from which nearly
all of us suffer at one time or another of our evils.

The question is naturally asked : To what is
this increase of nervous disorders due ? Most
people will agree that it is largely due to the
advance of civilisation ; to the wear and tear,
worry and anxiety of modern life ; to the break-
neck race for wealth, place and power, the
increased luxury and the struggle to maintain
appearances ; to the custom of working at high
pressure, the intense competition in all pursuits,
and the feverish activity of life in general. Not
only are we always in a hurry, but we should
be ashamed to admit that it was otherwise.
Our haste is further increased by the greater
rapidity of communication, and such factors as
steam, electricity, telegraph and telephone.
Then the roaring traffic grates on our nerves, if
not consciously, at least unconsciously. All this
tends to undermine nervous stability.

It is true that the modern apparatus of
civilisation, mechanical, hygienic, political, has
done much to diminish or even to abolish the
graver hazards of life and the ruder calls upon
our physical energy, and that upon the whole
it is both labour-saving and life-saving. Take,

for example, the telephone or the frequent letter
deliveries in our cities. They certainly make
intercourse between man and man easier in
respect of any one communication. But a
result is the multiplication of acts of communication. Every day the modern business man
has more numerous and quicker dealings than
he used to have. On each dealing there is a
saving of time and trouble, but may not this
be more than offset by the pace and variety of
mental adjustments involved in a day's work ?
The motor-car makes it easier and quicker for
a commercial traveller or doctor to go his rounds ;
but he can and does see more clients or patients
in a day, and thus the length of intervals and
the aggregate amount of rest as he moves from
house to house are reduced. The humble village
inhabitant has to-day a wider geographical
horizon, more numerous and complex intellectual interests than had the Prime Minister of a
petty State a century ago. If he but reads his
paper, let it be the most colourless provincial
rag, he takes part, certainly not by active
interference and influence, but by a continuous
and receptive curiosity, in the thousand events
which take place in all parts of the globe. A
cook receives and sends more letters than a
University professor did formerly, and a petty

tradesman travels more, and sees more countries and people, than did a reigning Prince of olden times.

All these activities, however, even the simplest, involve an effort of the nervous system and a wearing of the tissues. Every line we read or write, every human face we see, every conversation we carry on, every scene we perceive through the window of the flying express, starts into activity our sensory nerves and our brain centres. Even the little shocks of railway travelling, not perceived by consciousness, the perpetual noises and the various sights in the streets of a large town, our suspense pending the sequel of progressing events, the constant expectation of the newspaper, of the postman, or of visitors, cost our brain wear and tear.

Another cause for the increase of nervousness is the increased complexity of the brain as time goes on. The brain of the child, the idiot, or the savage is a simple organ compared with that of an adult of a civilised nation, and the complexity is ever increasing as the struggle for life becomes more severe. The march of education demands that more shall be learned, and competition on every hand and in every walk and calling perpetually urges men to fresh efforts and new paths of enterprise. Such increased complexity must as a matter of course lead to frequent disturbance of the brain and its functions. The adjustment between all the different relations and related parts must be easily put out of order, as in any very elaborate piece of machinery ; and, as in the latter, if the restoration is not speedily effected and the balance of the parts restored, the defect will increase and the machine will turn out bad work or no work at all.

As a rule, the active intellectual man is more readily apt to collapse under mental excitement than the individual of coarser fibre. The insensitiveness which belongs to the unintelligent is generally recognised. Savages are not troubled with nervous disorders, partly because their brain is less complex than that of civilised man and partly because they lead a simpler and more natural life.

The nervous tendency is becoming general. Many men are never really ill, nor well either ; that is to say, they are never ill enough to consult a physician, and never well enough to enjoy work or the pursuit of pleasure. In professional men the nervous tendency shows itself in alternating paroxysms of exaltation and depression, in oversensitiveness to criticism, and in premature breakdown. In business men it shows itself in "hustling," in the hurry to make money. Some people rush through life; it makes no difference where and when you meet them, they are always in a hurry. They make a great fuss, a big noise, and keep their mind and body working under a great strain. The nervous tendency reveals itself also in the morbid effusions of modern writers, whose principal themes are adultery, suicide and neurosis, and reflect the pessimism and morbid distortions of the modern mind. It shows itself in the decline of self-restraint, in the ambition of a very large section of the community to gratify its every appetite, satisfy its every whim, and obtain pleasure, and as much of it as possible, at any price and irrespective of all else. The unnatural and unwholesome desire to be regarded as "somebody" makes slaves of otherwise intelligent people and must be blamed for a great deal of our present-day unhappiness, heart-ache and sorrow. Their mind is ever filled with thoughts of discontent, because they do not possess wealth and the artificial prestige and power which are supposed to accompany riches. Thousands of men labour under the lash of debts and mortgages for no other reason than that they may enjoy the delusions of luxury. The idea that one must have fine clothes, diamonds, or automobiles, in order to maintain his place in society, has wrought the ruin and compassed the downfall of many otherwise happy families.

The "nervous" temperament predominates. It enables men to work more, but it also renders them more apt to exhaust their reserve force. Even if a man of nervous temperament is idle, the activity of his brain does not necessarily cease; only, its energy, having no proper outlet, will be turned inward and lead to self-observation and introspection. I have seen patients with well-developed brains and especially large frontal lobes who had never been trained to use their dormant capacities. Having no need to work for a living, or their occupation being too simple to engross their attention, they became victims of self-contemplation and suffered from various nervous ills. There is only one remedy for such men, and that is interesting pursuits. If useful interests were gained in early life such men would be saved from the peevishness, irritability and hypochondriasis of later years.

The large head is not always of an intellectual type, frequently the constitutional predisposition is of an emotional character. Such men have strong affections as a rule; they lack the power to be indifferent; they take things to heart easily. They are sensitive, frequently over-conscientious and lacking in self-confidence. They dwell more on their shortcomings than on their good qualities. Now, the effect of emotions is that they disturb the functions of the various bodily organs, temporarily only, it is true; but the man of nervous temperament is given to self-observation and is readily addicted to auto-suggestion, and both these factors help to make the disturbed function more or less permanent.

Doubtless one can say that in most cases of nervous disturbance many causes co-operate, and that if we examine individual cases we shall find that the most important of these causes is usually an inherited tendency; but this pre-disposition has only too often been fostered by faults in education and training in childhood, an education which has neglected the inculcation of self-control, self-denial and the habit of taking a healthy and kindly interest in every-thing and everybody.

A sound brain and nervous system rarely suffer from overwork, unless the work is done badly. The healthy adult brain is capable of doing much more work than it generally does do. There are few brains that are worked to their utmost, and nervous disorders are rarely, if ever, produced by regular and sustained labour, where the supply of force and power is equal to the demand. Fatigue is really very rare, transient and accidental in the case of men whose thinking is productive and fertile. On the other hand, it is very common and almost chronic among those who let life conquer them, among inactive men of meditative but non-productive brains, and even among those few men of real talent, who work only when inspired, work by spurts, so to speak, and then indulge in long periods of repose.

Many of the exhausting neurotic and psycho-neurotic affections are due to the failure of hard-worked men to secure such mental relaxation as will permit complete repair of nervous waste. Some men never get completely away from the set of thoughts with which they are occupied in their respective vocations. Waking or sleeping these thoughts are with them. Even when they try to turn to something else, their mental activity continues in the old groove to some extent, and so prevents the rest that is necessary for the repair of tissue. Under these conditions *re-creation* does not take place quite so well as it should, and even sleep does not relieve them from the burden of their mental work.

Some men through stress of business neglect

Nature's laws; they become careless about
their mode of living, neglect to care sufficiently
for their body, are careless about their meals,
shun exercise and recreation, " burn the candle
at both ends " ; all for the sake of their work.
Their only thought is for their work. No wonder
they break down in health. What would not
have worried them before does so now ; what
before was natural manly anxiety becomes restless uneasiness, perhaps even actual depression ;
they become apprehensive and irritable ; their
digestion is disturbed and sleep prevented until
they are totally unable to attend to their
work.

Intellectual work alone is one of the least
formidable causes of nervous exhaustion. The
man who attends to his duties free from worry,
anxiety, or other depressing emotions is not
likely to fall a victim to nervous exhaustion.
If he brings too lively an ardour to his work, or
if he prolongs his exertions beyond measure,
the result will be a state of fatigue more or less
profound according to the degree of resistance
of his brain, and nothing more. Fatigue and
the embarrassment of cerebral activity that
follows it will, of themselves, put an end to this
over-pressure, or will at least restrain it within
just bounds ; the nervous exhaustion that may

result from it will in such a case be speedily
reparable.

The great majority of those who suffer from
nervous exhaustion are people who are unable
to do things that they have to do. As a rule,
people do not become nervous wrecks while
they are succeeding; but they go to pieces
when they begin to fail. They begin to worry
and they go down. The human mind can accomplish wonders in the line of work, but it is soon
wrecked when directed in the channels of worry.
The brain-work that over-drives and exhausts
is that which accompanies care for the morrow,
worry caused by the end to attain, or fear of
failure, whether the matter at issue be one of
industrial or commercial affairs in which the
fortune is engaged, or one of an examination or
competition on which the future depends. We
wear ourselves out, not by hard work, but by
anxious thought regarding the adjustment of
work, and by nervous irritation at the failure
to accomplish an impossible task. Work and
worry are closely allied. Worry and anxiety are
common in this age of stress and competition.
Worry means a harassing preoccupation with
matters upon which no amount of taking
thought can be of the slightest avail, and often
with regard to questions which are not deserving

of the anxiety bestowed upon them. Worry means emotional strain, and emotions are not limited to the brain, but affect the bodily organs as well; that is why worry, anxiety, fear, disappointments, remorse, in a word, all states of sorrow and disquiet, exhaust the nervous energy.

No kind of psychic activity can be so persistently followed as worry. A fit of anger exhausts itself in a short time. Concentrated intellectual work reaches the fatigue point after a few hours. But worry grows by what it feeds on. One can worry more and worry harder on the fourth day than one can on the first. Every normal activity is strangled by it. The effects of overwork uncomplicated by worry are soon removed by rest; but rest from work thus complicated only redoubles the worries, the doubts and the scruples, gives rise to insomnia and thus causes additional damage.

When a strong and active mind breaks down suddenly in the midst of business it is worn out by worry rather than overwork. Work never killed a man, but worry drives many thousands of men and women to early graves. Worry exercises its influence upon man with a demon-like subtlety; it destroys his elasticity of gait; it contracts and narrows his normal breadth of intellect; it creates an atmosphere of misery in

which all things are contorted ; it robs life of
all its brightness, its pleasures, and its charms.
Worry is a cause of nervous exhaustion, and the
man or woman suffering from nervous exhaustion
worries on account of their worry. In other
words, they magnify trifles until they really
assume proportions of importance ; in fact, they
make mountains of molehills. They are given
to introspection, retrospection and apprehension.

Some people are born worriers. Their minds
are engrossed with small points that irritate
them, or filled with apprehensions of what is
about to go wrong. Folks are constantly looking
for trouble, crossing bridges before they come
to them, and one happy disappointment never
teaches them its lesson ; they go on worrying
just the same. Constantly regretting the things
that they have not done in the past, they brood
over their failures and look forward with dread
to that which may be, but very often is not.
The dread of adversity constantly imposes
numerous restrictions upon their enjoyment of
the present hour, and the calamities which never
happen and the griefs which never befall them
are perpetually casting shadows across their
sunniest paths. It is, indeed, the insane cultivation of the garden of trouble which brings to
them so bountiful a crop of the minor ills of life,

and which renders their minds and bodies weak
and fretful.

Some people are worried by a haunting
memory or remorse of some past failure, sickness,
or loss of property ; in some, the cause may be
found in the suppressed memory of a disagreeable experience making mischief without conscious knowledge of the person. Others are so
organised that there is frequent cause for
conflict between "the flesh and the spirit,"
that is to say, between the instinctive desires
and the moral nature. When a conflict occurs
between the repressed instinct and the conscious
mode of life, a neurosis or psychosis is liable to
develop. Again, in some we find a wrong
method of thinking, a point of view mentally
false or inadequate, or a careless allowance of
unwholesome mental moods, i.e. uncontrolled
emotions. True, no man is responsible for the
random thoughts that come flitting in and out
and the sensations which arise in him spontane-
ously, but we are all responsible for the thoughts
and feelings we deliberately entertain, hold and
dwell on.

All anxious emotions, if too long indulged in,
have the effects of lowering the health and
weakening the mental control. If any one be
subjected, for example, to adverse circumstances

for any length of time, to business worry or strain, financial difficulties or the never-ceasing worry of an unhappy domestic life, the strong, stable, healthy-minded man will remain that no longer. He has acquired just those conditions which are apt to cause nervous breakdown. Thus overwork, mental strain, grief or shock, when they do not in themselves produce disorders, may contribute to their development by lowering health and weakening mental control, and then the man of average mental stability passes into the second grade and becomes the man of neurotic temperament. The nutrition of the nerve cells has been deranged and they recruit their exhausted energy with increased difficulty. They no longer accumulate to the same degree as in health the force that they discharge; and there ensues a chronic enfeeblement of nerve strength, a nervous weakness and exhaustion. This state of exhaustion of the nervous centres produces conditions that are favourable to the development of a pathological mental state of depression, irritability, loss of will power, morbid fears and obsessions.

By worrying, we raise the blood pressure and hinder still further the proper working of the intellect, which is largely dependent on the maintenance of a well-balanced circulation

through the brain, and this in turn is dependent
not only on certain physical conditions, but also
on the state of mind. The care-free and the
joyous are able to do a vast amount of brain
work, experiencing but little mental fatigue;
whereas the victims of worry and grief, and
similar unhealthy mental states, find themselves
on the verge of brain-fag after engaging in the
most ordinary mental activities.

Most people try to overcome worry by simply
resisting it, thereby increasing it many times.
They would find that much more good can be
accomplished by surrender than by resistance
to it. If irritating or annoying memories,
or thoughts of any kind, are in any way awak-
ened, we should try to ignore them, not mind
them, and they will fade away. A large percentage of those things which harass and vex
us are robbed of their power if we but become
thoroughly reconciled to their presence. It is
our perpetual resistance that gives them such
great power to disturb us. If we do not mind
the source of the worry, we cease to fear it, and
the intellect will find means of conquering it
without the embarrassment of an emotion
which only hinders it. Forethought is an
intellectual force highly necessary to the smooth
running of our daily affairs; while fear thought,

anxious thought, is an emotional hindrance
wholly unnecessary and even highly injurious.
Instead of resistance we must try to direct our
attention away from ourselves. The best thing
is to get up and do something, or to get out and
see something. We should get up some hobby
to secure a diversity of interests. We should
be philosophical, enjoy the present, enjoy things
as we go along, live only one day at a time.
There is no need to live our whole past through
every day. Most of our worries are due to a lack
of confidence in our own ability, to a sense of
past failure and of future impotency ; hence it
is necessary to teach the man who worries how
again to become confident and self-reliant.

It will be seen that in our search for mental
causes we must be as conscientious as we are
accustomed to be in our physical investigations.
We must search the mind of the patient for the
source of his discomfort in exactly the same
spirit as we search the body for physical discomfort. We shall generally find some unhealthy mental states, such as depressive
emotions, apprehensions and fears, illogical
doubts and scruples, habits of morbid introspection and self-consciousness, derangement of
moral perspective, excessive concentration of the
attention on particular organs, and so on,

C

A frequent sign of nervous breakdown is that people do not heed the signs of fatigue produced by overwork or excessive worry, but fly to stimulants—alcohol, tea, coffee, or drugs—and with their pernicious aid suspend the warning signal of exhaustion. Unquestionably, alcohol is frequently taken by hard-working men to remove the sense of fatigue and to "oil the wheels of business," and what is most disastrous of all—to enable the worker to overwork himself. Thus many men become addicted to alcohol or drugs, and such a habit, when once established, produces a fresh series of nervous symptoms.

As our strongest passions and emotions are those connected with the sexual organs, it is not surprising that we frequently find the predisposing or exciting cause of a nervous disorder in sexual habits and the emotions associated with their activity. Excessive sexual indulgence, natural and unnatural, leads to nervous disorders ; on the other hand, sexual symptoms are apt to appear in persons suffering from nervous exhaustion, causing the patient still further distress. Sometimes there is only a lack of desire, but more often there is actual loss of potency, and sexual hypochondriasis is very common. These patients feel that they are losing virility or they dread the loss of it, and often fall into the hands of quacks who support their fancy. Some of them attribute the troubles with which they are afflicted to the habits which they practised in youth, especially when at school. They have often got this idea from the numerous books that are published on this subject by well-meaning but incompetent people or by charlatans. Whatever the cause, these symptoms usually disappear and potency is restored with the improvement in the nervous energy of the patient by appropriate constitutional treatment.

Nervous symptoms are also common when men approach middle age and, like women, undergo the " change of life."

Sometimes nervous disorders develop in people predisposed to them under the influence of a sudden fright, such as the mental shock caused by railway accidents. Generally speaking, shock is a state due to a sudden exhausting or depressing influence for which the individual is usually unprepared. This state of preparedness, that is to say, the attitude of the individual so far as expectation is concerned, is very important. It is a somewhat curious fact that many persons engaged in occupations or exposed in ways fraught with more or less likelihood of danger rarely suffer from nervous troubles, while those who are unconscious of any impending injury succumb at once upon its happening. Statistics show that there is a comparative absence of nervous disorder among those who are on the look-out, or who are consciously " taking their chances." It is also a noteworthy fact that the amount of fright and shock is often disproportionate to the degree of danger experienced.

Curiously, among middle-aged men it is not only the man who has led an exciting life, full of anxiety and worry, who is apt to break down, but sometimes men begin to ail from similar symptoms who have led a quiet and humdrum existence. The monotony of the lives they lead year in, year out, doing practically the same kind and amount of work without much variation, eating the same kind of food, from day to day, living in the same house and rooms without the slightest change even in the arrangement of the furniture, the same friends, often anything but stimulating in their conversation—causes the nervous system to revolt against all this monotony and symptoms of a nervous breakdown appear. Such men readily get well if a " change " is ordered, a change of air, a change of scene, of diet, and of company. All men who have to sit at desks doing the same kind of uninteresting work all the year round, and year after year, are subject to this form of disorder, unless they take care to have some interests besides.

Other abnormal modes of life—such as continuous confinement in bad air, unhealthy occupations, bad dwellings, faulty nutrition, and everything in general that reduces a person's general health and disturbs digestion and nourishment—make the nervous system less capable of resistance.

Anæmia, exhausting diseases, syphilis, influenza and malaria often lead to nervous disorders owing to changes in the blood causing defective nutrition of the nerve centres, thus diminishing their resistance and rendering them more vulnerable. Further, the altered secretions and excretions of certain cells and organs of the body circulating in the blood-stream influence the nerve centres and, in addition, certain abnormal chemical messengers—toxins—when present in the blood, are able to produce painful irritation of the nerves, while others produce fatigue, mental lassitude and despondency.

Many of the nervous disturbances described in this book are usually put under two headings. One is—

NEURASTHENIA, by which is meant an exhaustion of nervous energy giving rise to fleeting pains, abnormal sensations, mental instability, moral vacillation, constant worry, and most characteristic of all, a chronic sense of fatigue which is not relieved by either rest or sleep. The other is—

PSYCHASTHENIA, by which is meant a form of nervous exhaustion which is largely, if not wholly, due to psychic disturbances, the physical state of the patient having but little to do with the prevailing nervous weakness, loss of mental energy, fears, dreads, obsessions and melancholic tendencies.

This work not being intended as a textbook, I have not made use of these terms, and there are other reasons why I have omitted them. Both these terms are made to include an ever-increasing range of symptoms, some of them identical in both disorders ; neither do they constitute separate diseases in the sense that there is a distinct treatment for each. A man may have any of the symptoms of neurasthenia and not be a neurasthenic ; and the same is true of psychasthenia, which literally translated means psychic exhaustion, which is inconceivable. Debility of the nervous centres, on the one hand, and unhealthy mental states, on the other—such as wrong thinking, evil mental habits and unwholesome mental moods—can bring about functional disorder of any organ of the body through the nerves which connect it with the brain and spinal cord. As a rule they occur both together, one induced by the other, for which reason the general term PSYCHO-NEUROSES is frequently used ; and health cannot be regained until the nervous energy has been restored and healthy mental states substituted for the unhealthy ones. For these functional troubles there are no specific remedies. *We must treat the patient*, not alone his disorder. This is the principle which I have followed in my practice and which forms the basis of this work.

CHAPTER II

MENTAL SYMPTOMS OF NERVOUS EXHAUSTION .

LOSS OF MENTAL ENERGY, MEMORY AND
WILL POWER. FITS OF DEPRESSION

ONE of the commonest symptoms of nervous
disorder is weakness. Patients complain that
the least exertion, whether mental or physical,
produces an inordinate sense of fatigue. Lassitude is constant and hinders the commencement
of any activity, renders its execution painful,
and is so little mitigated by rest that it is by no
means uncommon to hear patients complain
that they are as tired after a night's rest as when
they went to bed.

A tired feeling is a prominent symptom of
nervous exhaustion. The first sign is usually a
feeling of undue weariness after moderate or
even slight exertion. Gradually all activity becomes painful. The patient cannot read without
becoming tired, nor listen to a conversation of
any length ; still less can he write, or apply
himself to any other work. He feels vague

24

diffuse pains, his appetite becomes languish-
ing, sometimes he grows thin, but often
enough he keeps his flesh and has an
illusory appearance of relatively good health.
He may be well nourished, muscularly well
developed, have had no immediate prostrating
illness or shock, nor has he been called upon
to bear any strain which ought not to have been
compensated for by appropriate rest and change ;
yet he is conscious of a want of brain tone,
sluggish action of mind, and of a deviation from
his normal condition of intellectual acuteness,
activity and vigour. His conviction of fatigue
exaggerates still more the fatigue itself. True
fatigue is doubled by the auto-suggestion of
fatigue ; it is aggravated by the emotional
fatigue from thinking about it.

Mental fatigue depends to a large extent on
the condition whether one is emotionally preoccupied or not. When the mind is peaceful the
nerve units are able to carry out their work
with the expenditure of a minimum amount of
energy; but when we are emotionally preoccupied,
working with a feeling of anxiety, anticipating
a possible difficulty, the work will be fatiguing.
Another fatiguing distraction is the habit acquired by so many nervous people of watching
themselves while they do their work, when the

very attention they bring to bear upon the effort that they are making is sufficient to hinder the action which they wish to perform. It is simply a case of the intervention of psychic phenomena which are focussed upon an act which, to be performed under the most favourable conditions, ought to be in some degree automatic. Again, many of these patients are constantly telling people they are tired and worn out, and they are everlastingly telling the same thing to themselves, little dreaming that this very contemplation and reiteration of their feelings is directly adding to the sum of their fatigue. If they were to accept their fatigue as a matter of course they would find that rest would soon cure it. They must learn not to emphasise their fatigue, or to magnify their weariness, by undue contemplation.

If the patient does not recover from his fatigue, he soon becomes painfully sensible of feeling mentally below par, and recognises his inability to use efficiently his powers of mind. He suffers from a torpid state of intellect, a mental malaise unfitting him for any kind or degree of cerebral work. The effort to think is irksome and painful, causing, if persevered in, dizziness, headache, painful confusion of thought and mental depression. The patient complains of an incapacity to control and direct the faculty of attention. He finds that he cannot, without an obvious and painful effort, accomplish his usual mental work, read or master the contents of a letter, newspaper, or even a page or two of his favourite book. The ideas become restive, and the mind lapses into a flighty condition, exhibiting no capacity for steady continuity of thought. The patient has so little control over his ideas that in his speech he, so to say, "runs off the lines" by introducing a great number of non-essential accessory ideas, which both obscure and delay the train of thought, and he needs to be frequently led back to his subject.

Confusion of thought is extremely common, that is to say, a state of mind in which there appears to be a flow of disconnected and incongruous ideas, and in which the flow of language, at any rate, is disconnected and incoherent. The confusion is due to a functional weakness in the logical combination and association of ideas, as a result of which the threads of thought are continually broken, the train of thought rendered imperfect, and often totally unrelated ideas are admitted into the mind.

The power of attention is weakened and the memory either wanders or is inconsistent in its associations. The patient is inattentive from sheer lack of power of application and mental endurance. He sometimes reads whole pages without having understood what he has read. Fully recognising his impaired and failing energies, he repeatedly endeavours to conquer the defect, and, seizing hold of a book, is resolved not to succumb to his sensations of intellectual incapacity, physical languor, and cerebral weakness. In his attempt to comprehend the meaning of the immediate subject under contemplation he reads and re-reads with a determined resolution, and an apparently unflagging energy, certain striking passages and pages of his book, but without being able to grasp the simplest chain of thought or follow successfully an elementary process of reasoning ; neither is he in a condition of mind fitting him to comprehend or retain, for many consecutive seconds, the outline of an interesting story or narrative of facts. Hence, after a time, only that which can be followed without an effort is welcome.

In this condition of nervous exhaustion the invalid is incapable of exercising continuity of thought for any lengthened period, and at times he is quite unable to think at all. This mental prostration disqualifies him for any occupation requiring the active use of the intellectual powers. He throws aside his favourite books, and even the newspapers, formerly a source of so much pleasure, become devoid of interest and distasteful. He neglects his ordinary vocation, feeling in mind blasé and able only to sit quietly in a state of mental abstraction or saunter about in a condition of gloomy reverie.

In this state of nervous ill-health serious injury is occasionally done to the delicate organisation of the brain by injudicious attempts to exercise, stimulate and force into activity the morbidly flagging and sluggish mental faculties. But the appearance of such symptoms indicates that the brain, although not in any way diseased, is quite unfit for any degree of sustained action, and that perfect repose and periods of prolonged and uninterrupted rest are necessary to a restoration of its enfeebled energies.

The faculty of memory is not infrequently impaired owing to the power of attention being diminished. The loss of memory extends, in well-developed instances, to an inability to recall proper names, dates, even single words. Without attention there can be no memory. The power of recalling past events becomes defective because these patients are unable to sustain the effort of attention necessitated by the search

for the forgotten incident, and because the
greater number of the events that have taken
place after the onset of their malady have been
perceived by them feebly, and hence are badly
associated with their conscious personality.
Often beset by some fixed idea, some hypochondriacal preoccupation, they live, so to speak, in
a state of perpetual absent-mindedness ; this is
one of the causes that makes them perceive in
a vague and uncertain manner the incidents of
which they are witnesses. Thus they are unable
to recall events to their memory even when they
are still recent.

Apprehensiveness, which is natural to all of
us, becomes greatly exaggerated. There are
persons who manifest the emotion of anxiety
upon the least pretext, and from this morbid
susceptibility arises a nearly constant state of
uneasiness. They are subject to doubts, hesi-
tations, fears concerning the most ordinary
circumstances and acts of life, because they
become quite incapable of willing effectively.
Some of these patients are congenitally apprehensive ; in others, an exaggerated apprehensiveness is acquired by habits which lower the
tone of the nervous system. They not only
lose initiative, the power to undertake new
enterprises, but they find it difficult to make up

their minds as to details of the ordinary affairs of life. These patients say that they cannot do things, their friends say "they will not," and the physician, taking the middle course, which, as usual in human affairs, has much more of truth than either of the extremes, says "they cannot will." There is an inability to "make up the mind," to come to a decision, to exercise a choice. This morbid perplexity of the intellect expresses itself in the actions. The patient no longer dares to do anything without endless precautions. There is a condition of doubt and an irresolution which is nearly always shown about the simplest details of everyday life. The patient is in a condition of constant hesitation from the most trivial motives, with inability to reach any definite result. He will hesitate a long time before he is able to decide whether to put on the right boot or the left, which foot to begin with in going upstairs, which pen to select out of a tray, what word to use to express his meaning, whether to walk this way or that, whether to take a stick or an umbrella. If he writes a letter, he reads it over several times for fear he may have forgotten a word or offended against orthography. If he is locking a door, he verifies several times the success of his operation. He worries usually over such trifles as whether he stamped a letter before posting it, whether it was properly addressed, whether he left a certain door open, or closed another door, whether a gas-jet is thoroughly turned off, a clock wound, and so on. And when, after numerous doubts and questionings and prolonged vacillation, a decision is reached, the sufferer finds little or no satisfaction in it, feeling certain that a different course should have been chosen. This propensity for doubting is absolutely unbounded. The patient is never certain of anything except that he is the most afflicted of mortals. This doubt and the indecision result directly from over-conscientiousness. It is because of an undue anxiety to do the right thing, even in trivial matters, that the doubter ponders indefinitely over the proper sequence of two equally important, or unimportant, tasks. When a patient has reached this stage he requires proper psychic treatment. He must be taught mental discipline and must be supplied with fresh motives for action drawn from those dispositions of his character which are elevating and healthy, but have been neglected by him. The treatment must be individual and may be helped by complete diversion of mind, serious occupation, and the cultivation of larger interests.

Sometimes such a patient will for ever ask questions, especially about his ailment. If he is not interrogating himself he is perpetually questioning others. He must know the how, wherefore, and why of everything. Every answer he receives is met by further questions, so that he becomes a nuisance if not an embarrassment to everybody with whom he comes in contact. If such a patient is much to be pitied, those who have the care of him are hardly less so. The need of reassurance leads him incessantly to question the people around him. In spite of formal affirmation, doubt arises each moment in his troubled mind; and he will reiterate during whole hours the same questions which reiterated and varied replies will never satisfy. His ailment is a subject of which he never wearies, sometimes the only one on which he can converse. He will return to it again and again with the same person, feeding his hopes on the same assurances and consoling himself with the same sympathies.

Mental irritability is another common condition, and is evinced more frequently in a man's domestic circle than in any other sphere. He frets and worries and becomes ill-tempered and even passionate over mere trifles, which, under normal conditions, would pass his observation

D

without special notice. He who is dissatisfied with himself is always more disposed to quarrel with others. The patient may get so fidgety and restless, rushing about, worrying everybody and fussing around until his friends dread the sight of him. He requires the attention of the entire household, and his shifting moods keep everybody about him in a mingled state of anxious solicitude and justifiable resentment. He finds it hard, even as a muscular manifestation, to evolve a smile and, except on very rare occasions when he momentarily forgets himself, he never makes the attempt. Tears, however, are always close to his eyes, ready to flow on every possible occasion—with one exception; the view of his own household, reduced by his conduct to weeping, leaves him with eyes as dry as parchment

Irresolution, hesitation, and the general enfeeblement of the will-power react upon the character. Such a person cannot meet the ordinary ills of life with a normal degree of fortitude; he grows discouraged with the smallest failures, magnifies every obstacle and professes inability to surmount it; he creates painful emotions by representing to his mind ideas of danger or of evil, or fear. He seems incapable of looking at questions calmly. Slight troubles and indispositions affect him seriously, and grave ones often cause profound depression. He makes mountains out of molehills, then toilfully climbs these self-created mountains, when clear-eyed reason would discover that the mountain needs no climbing, being only a mole-hill.

Even the most trivial of the routine tasks before him assumes portentous proportions, and anything out of the ordinary seems to him impossible of accomplishment. His motto is: " Never do to-day what you can avoid entirely or put off indefinitely." Consequently, to his detriment, financially and otherwise, he postpones important engagements and seldom forces himself to a decision in matters of moment. Particularly is this true of engagements at a distance. At the mere thought of their fulfilment he grows sick with apprehension; the actual fulfilment is downright agony. First come the terrors of the departure—the noise, bustle and confusion of the railway station. Then, with the journey actually begun, comes the realisation that every turn of the wheels is taking him further and further away from the only place in which he feels at all comfortable, namely, his home. At this he tries to divert his mind by reading, but finds his attention divided. What if anything should happen to him in his present situation ? This thought sets him quaking with dread, and he tries in a variety of ways, but with indifferent success, to banish it from his mind. At the end of the journey he is absolutely exhausted, and groans in spirit at the thought that his mission is yet to be accomplished. He wishes himself safely at home again, but pulls himself together as best he can to face the existing situation. What he suffers in mind and body during his stay is more easily imagined than described. It is enough to say that he does not know a happy moment until he finds himself back again at his original starting-point.

The patient is easily discouraged, shy, timid and fearful, and has lost confidence in himself and his own ability. He awaits with apprehension the outcome of every act, and doubts its justification and fitness. There develops a self-torture and an exaggerated feeling of liability. The ego will often become intensely exaggerated, and although the patient may be diffident in manner, still he is extremely self-conscious and shy, and he often labours under the idea that, whether at a party or in the street or at any place of public amusement, he is the observed of all observers. Walking up the gangway of a theatre or across a large room where people are sitting round, or being singled out for conversation at a dinner-party amid expectant silence, is a terrible ordeal to him. Whatever is said, done or left undone by others is analysed with reference to its bearing on himself. If others are indifferent it depresses him, if they appear interested they have an ulterior motive, if they look serious he must have displeased them, if they smile it is because he is ridiculous. That they are thinking of their own affairs is the last thought to enter his mind. It is hard for him to realise that the general gaze has no peculiar relation to himself. He often becomes over-conscientious and distresses himself needlessly with worries about business or family matters. He neglects his social duties, deliberately retires into solitude, and declares himself unable to manage his affairs. By the time this stage is reached the sufferer has become a consummate egotist. He has a deep-rooted conviction that nobody else in the wide world ever was or ever could be so afflicted. There are spells of more or less intense depression, and often the unreasonableness of these is appreciated by the individual, but he cannot rid himself of his morbid feelings. He now suffers from melancholy, but he is not insane, for however convinced of his trouble he is still looking for sympathy and possible help ; whereas the insane person, suffering from melancholia, is as a rule too downcast to care whether sympathy is offered or not, and would prefer death to cure.

Much depends on the reserve nervous force, the reserve energy, a man possesses. Persons in normal health, when they are tired, allow at times the dark curtain of discouragement to unfurl itself too far, but they regain control of themselves and soon recover their smiles, sometimes a little ashamed of the ease with which they have allowed themselves to be cast down ; whereas the man with little reserve nervous force who meets with a temporary trouble will drift into a condition of anxiousness and fear, and become depressed. It is toward the pessimistic side that he always leans. The slightest happenings are catastrophes for him, the smallest failures discourage him. He magnifies the obstacles which rise before him, and draws back at the sight of them. He is overcome by a telegram without having learned its contents ; he reads between the lines of a letter, and ascribes to any occurrence whatever the least probable and the most terrible causes. With him the dark curtain hangs very low, and he does not know how to raise it by a consoling reflection.

The habit of looking at the gloomy side of things is easily formed, and, once acquired, it becomes very forceful. Mental depression has a contracting effect on the personality, tends to keep the thoughts in one groove, on one set of ideas or objects, and that a narrow one. A patient in this condition is like a person living always in one small room with the blinds down : self-centred and miserable.

Nervous and sensitive people feel easily hurt and aggrieved and then their perception becomes so modified that they can see nothing on the brighter side of things. One may be dissatisfied, but one should not be discontented. All the world's progress is due to dissatisfaction with existing conditions and the putting forth of courageous efforts to improve the same ; all the sorrow of the world is born of discontent with our present circumstances. Psychic contentment is not incompatible with the highest degree of dis-satisfaction. Pessimism and optimism are largely a matter of habit. Normally, the mere process of living is of itself a positive delight, a continuous delight, and the smile with which we greet everybody and everything is not taught by convention. Misery is abnormal. Trouble does not actually exist. Trouble exists only in the fear thought of our own minds. We must

make a positive effort to extend the scope
of our mental action and think of things outside
of ourselves and our own interests. The attitude
of mind that should be cultivated is one in which
it is realised that, though there may be many
sources of evil in the world, there is a preponder-
ance of good even in the worst environment.
If there were no clouds we should not enjoy the
sun. Our happiness depends more on ourselves
than on circumstances. Opportunities for making
the best of things will be found by a cheerful
disposition. An excellent way is to try to cheer
up other people, if we cannot cheer ourselves.
After forgetfulness of self, the best cure is
thoughtfulness for others.

Much can be done for the relief of depression
by the influence of facial expression and bodily
attitude. If we assume a weak, slovenly carriage,
shuffling gait and inelastic step with the body
bent forward and insist on putting our features
into the shape which ordinarily expresses sadness, our attitude will be reflected internally,
and we shall become as sad as our expression.
On the other hand, if the features are drawn,
even by force of will, into the state that ordinarily
expresses cheerfulness and contentment, we
shall be tempted more and more to feel that way,
until at last even internal melancholy may be

dissipated. If a man throws back his shoulders, walks with a bold carriage and sure step, and takes in large breaths of air, expanding his chest and stimulating his circulation, his whole body as well as his mind feels the effect. Moreover, his associates will respond to the mood he is in, thus reinforcing his condition.

But it is not by advice alone, however excellent, that we shall get the patient well. We must first ascertain and remove the cause of the nervous exhaustion, which has given rise to the excessive fatigue and the mental symptoms of doubt, indecision, and depression, and restore the nervous energy, before we can appeal to the patient's reason with any hope of success.

CHAPTER III

LOSS OF MENTAL CONTROL.
OBSESSIONS AND MORBID FEARS

NERVOUS debility and exhaustion, if at all
protracted, is almost sure to produce a variety
of mental symptoms, nearly all of which are
due to one factor, weakening of mental control.
One of the commonest complaints is loss of
power to resist the invasion of certain ideas
that obtrude themselves upon the patient's
mind and, for the moment, completely occupy
it. They are recognised by him as being
foreign to his personality and his modes
of thought, and are not, at any rate in most
cases, blended with his individuality, but held
as unreasonable and morbid, by the patient
himself. They are simply ideas or feelings that
he cannot get rid of at the time. Practically
they are only exaggerations of the experiences
of most, if not all, normal individuals, and it is

only through the degree of this exaggeration that they carry their victims over the borderland of mental health.

Even normal persons sometimes are annoyed by some persistent idea, but the idea vanishes when not seriously entertained. The person, however, who is suffering from brain-fatigue or nervous exhaustion cannot shake off the obsessive idea, which may be either ideational or emotional.

The majority of IDEATIONAL OBSESSIONS are harmless and unattended by mental distress, or interference with health or occupation; but any of them may, if the nervous energy has been weakened, attain to such magnitude as completely to overwhelm and temporarily to cripple the subject. They do this not only by occupying all his attention by their prominence, but by destroying natural rest by their persistence, and by causing great distress if they are resisted; or, if uncomplied with, by producing remorse and agony of mind. Their fixity is recognised by the patients themselves as something clearly morbid, and they feel that it constitutes an obstacle to the normal course of ideas and actions, an extraneous element in the normal current of thought which no effort is able to dislodge. When the idea is in itself of trifling

importance, it is its fixity only which renders it
unpleasant. Probably the idea which is presented in an unusually insistent manner does
not assume the character of a fixed idea until
its particular insistence has become an object
of attention and a cause of uneasiness, and has
been rendered not only harassing but is also
feared. Such fixed ideas may consist of words,
numbers, phrases, or melodies, or there may be
obsessions of counting objects uselessly, repeating words of formulæ, of stepping in a certain way, of touching certain things in a regular
order, or uttering obscene words.

The EMOTIONAL OBSESSIONS are more fixed
and more serious. They are generally based on
memories of a disagreeable character, of which
the details may be forgotten, but not the event
itself. We often remember against our will
matters that we would rather forget. Such
capacity to forget painful experiences differs
greatly in different people and is greatly
diminished when the nervous system is debilitated. Not only are emotional obsessions distressing in themselves, but they are accompanied
by a disagreeable form of emotion, generally
that of fear. Hence the long list of "phobias,"
which include disgust, dread, or aversion, absurd
and unnatural, towards many things, harmless

and harmful. Such aversions are *claustrophobia*, the horror of being in an enclosed space ; *agoraphobia*, the horror of being in an open space ; *mysophobia*, the horror of uncleanliness, and so forth. In these cases there is a morbid and irrational horror which is well known by the subject of it to be morbid and irrational, but which yet dominates his conduct. Sometimes the natural repugnance associated with certain acts is enormously exaggerated ; thus there may be fear of contamination, of contagious diseases, of going into dangerous places. Or the fixed ideas consist in the representation of the impossibility of accomplishing certain acts, a representation which is translated into a real impossibility. Or they consist in the representation of involuntary phenomena, which, however, may actually take place through the simple suggestive effect of the representation, as in the fear of blushing or in obsessive insomnia. Or they may originate with some special experience ; an apparently narrow escape from being run over may be the inciting cause of a dread of crossing streets ; a sudden morbid impulse or suggestion to throw one's self down may be the cause of a phobia as regards all high places. Some unpleasant experience, or the mere reading of one in a sensational newspaper

paragraph, may give rise to the fear of being
alone, of sleeping alone in a room, or being left
alone in a railway compartment. In all cases,
it is the weakened inhibition that is at fault.
It is easy to see how almost any variety of obsessions of dread may thus arise, and most of
us can, from our own experience, appreciate
their possibility. Given the necessary susceptibility, circumstances doubtless dictate the
direction the phobia shall take.

As regards the agoraphobe and claustrophobe,
the fear of being in an open space or in an
enclosed space, as the case may be, is a derivative
of the instinct of self-preservation. This primi-
tive instinct prompts the aversion from all those
situations and circumstances which threaten
bodily injury. It gives rise to that indescribable
feeling of unpleasantness which most people
experience on looking down from a great height,
even though they may be quite efficiently
guarded from falling. There is no danger of
falling ; there is an insurmountable railing at
the edge of the precipice, which is manifestly
a completely efficient safeguard ; yet it is
impossible to approach the edge voluntarily, and
if we are compelled to approach the edge a
horrible feeling is experienced which cannot be
suppressed or reasoned away.

When persons afflicted with agoraphobia enter an open space, or pass through a street that is devoid of people, they are immediately overcome by the imperative idea of the impossibility of going on, and thus they become so anxious and nervous that they are actually paralysed ; while if they keep close to the houses or are accompanied by someone, they have no difficulty whatever. The painful situation in which the patient finds himself leads to anxiety and to physical manifestations, such as a rush of blood to the head, mental confusion and palpitation, as a result of which the painful feeling becomes still more intense. The patient recognises the absurdity of his dreads, and in a feeble way strives against them; but the lassitude of will is too great to be overcome and he returns to his fears and anxieties. The claustrophobe who is shut up in a railway carriage, or the agoraphobe who is in an open space, is as thoroughly and completely aware of his safety, and of the irrationality of his terror, as the person on the edge of the cliff who is safeguarded by a stout railing from falling over; but none the less is he incapable of utilising his knowledge to suppress his panic.

Another noteworthy example is the *fear of fire.* Both in his own house and in public

buildings the victim of this fear is at once thrown
into a panic by the faintest smell of smoke whose
exact origin he does not know. At home he is
unwilling to have even the tiniest fire burning
in a grate unless he can be present to keep an
eye upon it, and he never retires for the night
without assuring himself that the range and
furnace are in a perfectly safe condition. If he
plans to spend some time in an hotel he makes it
his first duty, after being shown to his room, to
acquaint himself thoroughly with the location
of the nearest fire-escape.

Frequently the dominant element is the *fear
of fainting* in a public place and the com-
motion that would follow such a mishap. The
sufferer, by his over-exalted powers of imagination, pictures to himself this scene in minutest
detail. In his mind's eye, he sees people crowding
about him, thrown into utmost confusion by
his plight; the uprushing ambulance with its
driver urging on his horse and sounding his
gong; and the casualty ward of a hospital with
its bustling attendants. His other senses rapidly
supply the remaining details of this picture,
which may come to his mind even when he is
sitting in the quiet atmosphere of the home and
produce an anguish of mind and body fully
equal to that experienced in the localities

mentioned. Thus a person may have a fear
of railway trains, of theatres, of church, of
crowded and solitary places, of social entertain-
ments, but in each of these it may be the same
and only fear—that of fainting ; just as another
person fears water, knives, fire-arms, high places,
and gas, when his real fear is suicide, these
objects being conceivable methods by which
suicide can be effected.

The patient resists, combats, represses, denies,
and fights his fixed ideas, and all the while his
mental warfare constitutes an ever-present
source of auto-suggestion which tends to grow
stronger and stronger. To overcome obsessions
by volitional effort, it is far better to make that
effort in the direction of thinking of other
subjects, or of doing some work that has nothing
to do with the obsession, than to " reason it out "
and make efforts of will directly in the teeth of
them. My advice to the victims of obsessions is
to disregard them, not to mind them, not to
fear them. It is the only way of getting rid of
them. Evade them rather than stand up to
them, should be the rule in most cases. Turn
into a side road rather than meet your enemy in
the face of his line of communication. Better
to switch the mind on to a loop line and let the
foe pass by. Singing or whistling to keep up

E

courage is no mere figure of speech. If at the same time everything possible is being done to improve the tone of the nervous system, the constitutional apprehensiveness will disappear and there will be less likelihood of a relapse.

Fixed ideas often lead to IMPULSIVE ACTIONS, due again to defective mental or emotional control. Some people naturally have little self-control, and that little has not been cultivated during their youth, so that it takes a small occasion for them to lose it. Every one of us has his brain traversed sometimes by foolish abnormal impulses, but these sudden and unusual conditions do not pass into action because they are bound down by a contrary force, an inhibitory will-power, which simple fatigue often renders unstable and precarious ; the will, we must remember, being the power not only to do something, but also to leave something undone.

A large number of people have impulses to perform useless, bizarre, and even dangerous acts. At certain moments they feel the desire for these actions arising in them. They are fully conscious of the absurdity of these actions and judge them at their true worth. There is more or less serious and real struggle between the tendencies which urge them on and the judgment which holds them back. Such people often resist when the act appears to them really bad ; they yield when, rightly or wrongly, they regard the act as of little consequence. The act once performed, the patient experiences a peculiar satisfaction, a feeling of relief, which is in turn followed by remorse for having committed it, should it be of an immoral or criminal nature, and often by a great anxiety, lest the obsession should again occur.

These impulses are as manifold in their form as are the obsessions of doubt or fear, and vary in their importance and severity from the simple easily rejected suggestion, as to say or do something wrong, to the most inconvenient or dangerous impulses to serious crimes, such as assaults, arson, suicide, or homicide. Many of these patients seek medical advice to counteract the obsession, for fear their dangerous impulses may be put into action.

Theft is very common. The article stolen is usually not made use of, or is replaced unawares. It is the shame of being regarded as a genuine thief that prevents a frank confession. The majority of patients, however, have only a " fear " of stealing when seeing valuables exposed ; they suffer agonies in consequence, but their impulse is successfully repressed.

I have seen patients who at the sight of knives were overcome by an impulse to kill someone, perhaps someone near and dear to them. Most of these patients knew that they were not likely to do anything silly or criminal, but they dreaded that they might do so one day and suffered intense agony in consequence. There was generally a history of nervous breakdown or of unwholesome habits which gradually lowered the nervous energy, on the restoration of which by appropriate treatment all these symptoms disappeared.

There are patients who come to the physician worked up because they fear they may commit suicide. Every now and then the thought comes to them that some time or other they will perhaps throw themselves out of a window, or be tempted to drop in front of a passing train, or over the side of a steamboat, or impulsively take poison. Some nervous people become quite disturbed by these thoughts. Their nervousness over the fear of this may serve to make them supremely miserable.

Very few men, shaving themselves with an ordinary razor, have not sometimes had the thought of how easy it would be to end existence by drawing the edge of the razor through the important structures in the neck. Now there are persons who at moments of worry and nervousness are so affected by this thought that they have to give up shaving themselves. Such patients need firm and convincing reassurance that there is no danger that they will commit suicide, because it is extremely rare that patients who dread it very much and, above all, those who dread it so much that they take others into their confidence in the matter, take their own lives. The very fact that the thought produces so much horror and disturbance in them is the best proof that they will not impulsively do anything irretrievable in this way.

Coming back to the discussion of morbid fears, their range is boundless. To enumerate them all would be an endless task. There is one form of fear which, however, merits separate consideration. It is the fear of sickness.

In some persons there is a MORBID ANXIETY AS TO HEALTH, and extremely exaggerated, if not illusory, ideas as to the existence of certain bodily disease, leading to the concentration of the attention upon, and consequent exaltation of, physical sensibility, resulting often from passing physical sensations or slight ailments, which eventually assume to the deluded imagination a grave and significant character. No part of the body is exempt from these fears, but usually the attention is centred upon the obscure and inaccessible organs. The patient may present the picture of health, or he may have some real ill regarding which he is unduly anxious. As a rule there is a retardation, if not inhibition, of the functional activity, a lowered tone, of that organ on which the patient's attention is concentrated and which he expects to go wrong. There is an apprehension or fear of disease, not a genuine conviction, hence the patient talks to everyone he meets about his ailments to get some further clues about their realities. At first he will be amenable to reason; but if not dealt with firmly and if the nervous disorder is not treated, which lies at the root of his trouble, his fear may give way to a decided belief, a fixed idea.

The subjects generally lead sedentary and solitary lives and their morbidity is often accentuated by reading quack literature. They show extraordinary pertinacity in seeking cures for their ailments. Nearly all of them complain either of actual pain or of some form of bodily discomfort. There is often a state of mental gloom and depression. They are apt to be irritable, emotional, restless, and sleepless. Their minds may be so occupied with their miserable condition that work, or even amusement, is quite out of the question.

We all of us get tired ; but we know what it is, and we are assured beforehand that a little rest is all that we need. The nervous person, however, is frightened ; he takes his weariness with great concern and makes it last longer by the attention that he pays to himself. The human mechanism is so complicated that hardly a day goes by without our noticing some creaking in the works. Sometimes it is gastric trouble, or a slight pain or palpitation of the heart, or a transient neuralgia. Full of confidence in our comparative health we keep right on, making light of these little ailments. Some persons, however, are fascinated by the idea of sickness ; it becomes a fixed idea with them.

A common, and at the same time, secretly nourished fear is *the fear of insanity*. The anguish occasioned by it is indescribable. This fear is caused in part by queer feelings in and about the head, in part by memory defects, and, lastly, by the unwelcome presence of whimsical ideas and constantly recurring impulses to do things which the sufferer recognises as entirely foreign to his normal self.

As a matter of fact there is not in these patients the profound alteration in character we are wont to observe in insanity. Intimate letters may be rambling, and overcharged with

petty details of distresses and incapacities, but
they do not betray aberration of mind, as those
of the insane almost invariably do. The insane
person, like one in a dream, is apt to be as un-
aware of his symptoms as the sufferer from
nervous exhaustion is morbidly alive to them. The
latter's mind may be occupied with his complaint
to the exclusion of some better thoughts and
impulses, but is rarely perverted or blinded.
He is certain that he is ill, and in his
belief he is justified, but he is always open to
argument as to the cause or seat of his discomfort, and his confidence is to be won. He
rarely loses hope entirely and seeks each new
physician with fresh prospects of relief. If he
is sad, his sadness is the natural event of baffled
hopes and thwarted enterprises. He may shun
society, but he does so only because conversation
wearies him and people get on his " nerves."
In his solitude and centred in himself he may
develop eccentric or crazy habits, but rarely
insanity.

The patient suffering from nervous exhaustion
wishes to make the effort to act, but he cannot,
fatigue setting in quickly. The insane patient
suffering from melancholia has no such wishes ;
he is indifferent towards everything and feels
as if paralysed. The mental depression of the

former is not immovable; under the influence of some stimulus, as that of enlivening society, he may recover at least temporarily. With the latter the gloom is constant. The former, as a rule, consults the physician of his own accord, desirous to get rid of his various symptoms. The latter rarely takes the initiative, but so alarms his family that it is they who consult the physician. The former is never without hope; the latter has no desire to live.

Another common fear is the fear of heart disease, with its popularly supposed termination in sudden death. Fear of cancer is also not uncommon. Others fear sexual disease or brood over what they regard as the penalty of youthful wrongdoing. Such patients are especially likely to become the prey of quacks, who levy heavy tribute on their unwholesome fancies.

The suffering of the world is out of all proportion to the actual disease. Many people who have little disease suffer a great deal, partly from over-sensitiveness, partly from concentration of mind on their ailments, and partly from such ignorance of whatever pathological condition is present that they grow discouraged and morbid over it. In such people a vicious circle is formed when anything is the matter. First they dread a particular illness. This keeps them

from enjoying life as before and they restrict
their activities. Perhaps they become over-
careful of their diet and reduce it below the
normal limit for healthy activity. This causes
them to have less energy for work and disturbs
their sleep. Then a host of minor symptoms,
supposed to be due to the disease, whatever it
is or they think it is, but really consequent upon
the unhealthy habits that have been formed,
begin to develop.

The patient may be merely " apprehensive "
about his health and be amenable to reason ;
he may let himself be convinced by arguments
when they are skilfully put before him. Such
patients may exaggerate the importance of their
symptoms and attribute them to an impossible
cause ; they are, however, quite willing to be
set right, and, once convinced of their error,
their suspicions may altogether vanish. Others
there is no need to convince that they are
deceiving themselves ; they know it as well as
their doctors do. It is rarely that they are under
any delusion as to the groundlessness of their
apprehensions ; much of their distress arises
from their being unable to control fears that
they realise are " foolish " ; they are disturbed
by it just as we sometimes are in ordinary life
at the thought of a danger that we know to be

chimerical. Others, again, are no longer beset by fears; they have true delusions, such as having cancer of the stomach or some other incurable complaint. They are not simply apprehensive, they are convinced; fear has given place to a decided belief, a fixed idea.

The rational treatment of morbid fears must be founded on a careful study of individual cases, the recognition of the special cause, a neutralisation of all unfavourable suggestions, and occupation of mind that will enable the patient to rid himself of the annoyance occasioned by them and the physical symptoms that so often develop as a consequence. The patient has to learn not to fear the intrusion of strange thoughts and feelings, to regard them with indifference. Being robbed of their significance they soon fade away and disappear altogether. Both dreads and obsessions require the practice of mental discipline and self-control; otherwise, even when the nervous system has been put right, the old mental habits will bring about another relapse. All such nervous sufferers will do well to take up new lines of study or new hobbies in order to think as much as possible of things outside of themselves and their own interests. They ought to observe others as much as possible and not themselves. As has been pointed out already, they should make a point of cheering up other people. Their good humour will act on them by reflection. Let them cultivate also the habit of contentment and avoid worrying over things which cannot be changed. A large percentage of the things which harass and vex us would be robbed of their power of annoyance if we became reconciled to their presence.

CHAPTER IV

INSOMNIA

AMONG the symptoms of nervous disorder there is one of great importance because of its frequency and the aggravation that it causes in the patient's condition. This is insomnia.

Sleep varies in degree and kind. It may be wanting altogether; it may be too short; it may be too prolonged; it may not be deep enough; it may be interrupted; it may be disturbed by dreams; it may be unrefreshing, or it may be too profound. Want of sleep will in time wear out the finest and strongest brain. All sorts of diseases result from want of sleep. Of course, as in everything else, the widest differences may be observed between one person and another in regard to the amount of sleep required. What is sleeplessness to one person may not be so to another. There are men who require not more than five hours' sleep, others must have seven hours regularly, and there are some who sleep nine hours and even more.

Much depends on the nature of the occupation and on habit; and there are in this matter, too, good and bad habits. The habit of sleeping too little is less frequent than that of sleeping too much. There are some hard brain workers who sleep very little and yet enjoy good health if they live otherwise correctly. This fortunate power of rapid recuperation may be said to be one of the characteristics of greatness. At all events, it has occurred with sufficient frequency in great and successful men to have done great harm among average individuals. No one ever got too much healthy, natural sleep. Some anæmic and nervous individuals recuperate with such extreme slowness that they require ten, twelve, or thirteen hours of sleep properly to redress the balance. As a rough working average it may be stated that the majority of vigorous adults require about seven hours' sleep. As a rule, it is not the length of sleep, but its quality which is at fault.

The majority of patients suffering from nervousness sleep badly, but their insomnia appears under very different forms. There are patients who get to sleep with difficulty. They go to bed tired, but when they are in bed sleep does not come. Certain patients fall asleep easily, but they wake up at the end of a few hours and cannot get to sleep again; many fall asleep toward morning at the hour when they ought to get up. Again, some describe their sleep at night as abnormally profound, but complain that they are so little refreshed by it that they remain drowsy and lethargic during the day, unable to attend to business. *Drowsiness* is the opposite condition to insomnia and is equally a sign of nervous exhaustion.

Many patients find their insomnia caused by various painful sensations, such as palpitations and anguish, or dyspeptic troubles. It seems to them as though they could go to sleep if they could be relieved of all these discomforts. Others sleep, but with agitated sleep, disturbed by dreams and nightmares. Sometimes they preserve no memory of the dream, but are conscious of having had an interrupted and disturbed sleep by their state of feeling in the morning.

Besides work and worry, the general rush of life of modern civilisation does not tend to healthful sleep. At the present day, when so many people, either from choice or necessity, spend their time in passing from one form of excitement to another, from work to play and play to work in a limited number of hours, and the nervous system is always in a state of

tension owing to newspapers, telephones, tele-
graphs and motor-cars, it is not to be wondered
at that sleeplessness is so common a trouble.
Then there are the traffic noises in town; and when
our nerves are upset by them and we seek the
quiet of the country or seaside we find that we
have become sensitive to the noises made by
dogs, birds, the rustling of leaves, or the beating
of the sea waves against the shore, noises of
which in perfect health we should have taken
no notice.

A clock that strikes the quarters has spoiled
many a night. To others, the mere ticking of
the clock is enough to keep them awake. Some
people are more sensitive to one kind of noise
than to another. Recurrent noises are the worst,
causing people to lie awake in the expectation
that they will recur.

Excess of light in a bedroom, such as proceeds
from a fire, or in summer from the early morning
light, often prevents sleep. Change of climate,
especially to high altitudes, or in some individuals even to the seaside, or sleeping in a
strange bed, sometimes gives rise to a temporary
insomnia. Eating late dinners or suppers by
those unaccustomed to them ; or the failure to
obtain the habitual " night-cap," whether it be
a glass of hot milk or something stronger, in

those accustomed to it, will delay sleep in others. As a rule, the generous feeders sleep better than the careful eaters, the continued congestion of the digestive organs depleting the brain and favouring sleep, provided no dyspeptic troubles arise.

Sleeplessness may arise in persons in health from keeping irregular hours. A rule that should be followed by everyone is to practise going to bed at a definite hour every night and to get up at a definite time every morning; moreover, to get up immediately on waking. Regularity in the habit of retiring is of more importance than going early to bed. All our functions are regulated by habit. We often have an appetite at the hour for dinner, even when we have not spent our strength or exhausted our capital, and when we have taken food a few hours before. Our eyelids grow heavy at the time when we habitually go to bed, although we have displayed no particular activity during the day-time; and by training ourselves to definite time for sleeping, and avoiding all exciting causes prior to going to bed, sleep is almost sure to come.

Regularity in the hour of rising should also be practised. Except invalids, no person should lie in bed during the morning hours when not

F

asleep. To those awakening in the middle of the night and unable to get to sleep again, I have advised getting up and doing some unexciting mechanical work for half an hour, rather than remaining fidgety in bed. Getting up under these circumstances soon produces a tired feeling, and the body being cooled a little, the warmth of the bed is again appreciated and sleep is more likely to follow.

Another good rule is to train one's self to fall asleep without delay immediately after retiring. We cannot sleep if we continue to think. In some people the thoughts are fixed on a disturbing subject ; some are kept awake by worry and fears, while others suffer from too vivid an imagination. The fancy, instead of becoming gradually subdued, until the supervention of unconsciousness, increases in activity ; while myriads of fantastic thoughts crowd upon the mind in endless procession and baffle every attempt at repose. During the early part of the night such persons lie awake for several hours, tormented by a constant succession of thoughts and emotions of the most varied character, and not till towards morning do they usually succeed in falling asleep. The patient must enforce upon his consciousness the fact that nothing can be gained by reconsideration of the sins of omission or commission in the hours past, or at least nothing so valuable that it should be allowed to lessen the period of needed rest. Though it is not easy to empty the mind, to stop its involuntary activity, the patient can train himself to replace the active labour of the mind with peaceful contemplation, to turn the thoughts into different channels. Sometimes this is best accomplished by physical means, sometimes by fixing the attention on merely idle but pleasant notions. Many active-minded people of intelligent habit find a dose of light literature a useful means of altering the current in which thought has been running, and read poetry or fiction before bed· time. But they should be careful not to get so interested that they keep awake to read. The book should not be so dull that it cannot be read at all ; on the other hand, it must not be exciting, or it will murder sleep.

There is one preoccupation which is especially dangerous ; it is that of sleep itself. There is ample reason to believe, and many cases support such a conclusion, that a great deal of the insomnia of nervous patients originates in, and is fostered by, an obstinate and continued belief that sleep is impossible. When the patient does not sleep and is impatient because he does not sleep, and keeps turning over and over, and growing more and more vexed, he creates a state of agitation which hinders sleep.

During the hours of insomnia the mental condition of the patient is very variable. I have seen some who do not suffer at all. They admit coolly that they do not sleep, but they do not experience any unpleasant sensation. Others become impatient and grow vexed. They turn over incessantly in bed, get up, and go back to bed again. They toss from side to side, remove the bedclothes, change their position continually in the vain endeavour to become unconscious. The peripheral nerve irritation occasioned by their contortions only serves to perpetuate the condition of cerebral wakefulness. When, as frequently happens, sleep at last supervenes, it is no longer physiological in character; but, on the contrary, is perverted by dreams and unconscious cerebration to such a degree that it affords little or no refreshment. Daylight finds these patients completely prostrated and unable to resume their accustomed activities with the requisite amount of energy.

As to dreams, all we can say of them is that they appear to be due, to put it crudely, to different areas of the brain or parts of the body varying in the degree of their fatigue and consequently soundness of their sleep. A study of a large number of the dreams which psychologists have analysed shows that the greater part of the material out of which the dreams are fashioned is furnished by the previous waking thoughts of the dreamer, particularly those disconnected ideas which coursed in a passive fleeting way through the mind, or rather which made up the stream of consciousness just before going to sleep. Another source of these dream elements —although a less rich one—is the thoughts of the preceding day, and even earlier mental experiences. The same might be said of ideas and feelings which had dominated the psychological life of the individual through a long period of time, and the subconscious mental experiences of which the individual is only dimly aware. There are a multitude of events which are so completely forgotten that no effort of the will can revive them, which may nevertheless be reproduced with vividness in our dreams. In the opinion of modern investigators, dreams are related mainly to dissociated, suppressed, or dormant past experiences, dormant wishes or desires, and originate chiefly in the subconscious mental life. In their opinion, the world of dreams is the embodiment of our hopes and fears. The thoughts which we recall on awakening are merely the manifest thoughts of the dream, but by a process of psycho-analysis we can get at the latent thoughts. The former are absurd and meaningless, while the latter are the actual innermost thoughts of the individual.

The troubled or horrid dreams which occur during sickness are probably due to the torturing of the brain by the toxins with which the blood is loaded. Similarly, the gruesome visions and nightmares which embitter the slumbers of those under the stress of violent emotions and mental suffering are due to similar action by the fatigue-poisons produced by these states.

While perfectly normal sleep is dreamless, yet a moderate amount of dreaming, especially if the images evoked are of a pleasing or indifferent character, is quite compatible with good and refreshing slumber. Persistent or frequent bad dreams are, like insomnia, a sign of ill-health, and should be regarded and treated as such.

Those patients who approach the night with a fixed idea that they will not sleep and who count the bad nights which they have already had, persuaded that this one will follow in line and resemble the others, should remember that the best preparation for sleep is confidence that one will sleep, and indifference if one does not. It is necessary for the patient to lose all fear of

insomnia and to approach the subject of sleep
with a perfect indifference, which may be
summed up in this idea : " If I sleep, so much
the better ! If I do not sleep, so much the worse,
but it does not matter either ! " Sleep comes
when one is not looking for it ; it flies away when
one tries to catch it. It may be pointed out to
these patients that it is a mistake to elevate
sleep into a fetish ; that the world does not
come to an end because one person, however
important, is unable to sleep ; and that the
most certain method of keeping such an elusive
entity from embracing one is in pity to implore
its advent with outstretched hands, or to summon
it peremptorily and impatiently with clenched
teeth.

In some persons thoughts keep on trooping
through the mind in a regular procession and
thus prevent sleep. Such persons, if they cannot
otherwise stop thinking on retiring, may achieve
success by allowing the train of thought to
march on with all its energy, while they begin
to concentrate the mind on relaxing the body,
when it will usually be found that the train of
thought slows down just in proportion as the
muscles are relaxed. Or else, if this fails, the
patient should try, as I have mentioned before,
to think of something pleasant and attractive,

but calm and reposeful. To the romantic, the
moonlight on a quiet sea may be suggested ;
to the more material, a comfortable armchair
in front of a fire ; but he must go on thinking
about it. He must concentrate all his attention
upon it, and must not be surprised if at first the
charm fails to work. When the attention tires,
a not too interesting book may be temporarily
appealed to, and then the experiment repeated.
If the patient can be induced to act thus for
several nights in succession without allowing his
thoughts to revert in pity to his sleepless state,
it is astonishing what success will often ensue ;
more especially if, by an appeal to his reason
and proper pride, one has succeeded in enlisting
his real co-operation.

The one procedure which most universally
disposes to sound sleep is one which is within
the reach of all, and that is getting well tired.

Another rule which I always impress upon
my patients is to have done with all serious
thoughts before entering their bedroom. None
but cheering and soothing reflections, if any,
should take place prior to going to bed. Any
topic which stimulates the brain to great
activity, whether intellectually or emotionally,
must be carefully excluded. There should be
a period of absolute quiet before retiring to bed

In order to sleep well patients must be thoroughly comfortable in bed. Most people find they sleep easiest with a reasonably firm pillow, not too low, so that the head is a little higher than the body ; others raise the head of the bed, so that there is a gentle slope. The lateral position is to be preferred to lying on the back. Sensitive persons sometimes obtain sleep by changing their position in bed, or, better still, the position of the bed. It is held by some of great importance whether the bed faces North, South, East, or West.

As regards the room to sleep in, a good bedroom should be spacious, not encumbered with furniture and draperies, since much fresh air is needed when sleeping. Active ventilation is not less necessary, and should be so arranged as to avoid currents of cold air; for the skin during sleep, in consequence of the increased perspiration, is very sensitive to cold, and the body is more easily chilled asleep than awake. The bed should therefore be placed near the inner wall, as far as possible from the windows and the fireplace, to avoid the draughts which are strongest at these spots. Some people sleep well when they have a change of room, and others when they have a change of air A holiday, with a complete change of scene and distinct change of activities, will often do much to cure insomnia.

Sources of local irritation must be removed. For example, where the feet are persistently cold, warmth may be applied to them. Sometimes a hot bath or hot sponging, followed by very gentle drying, will bring on sleep by allaying nervous irritability.

Diet has little influence on sleep, except when insomnia is due to disturbances of digestion. The processes of digestion probably go on more slowly during sleep, but they are perfectly carried out, as is illustrated by the almost invariable habit among animals of going to sleep directly after a meal. Indeed, a moderate amount of food in the stomach or intestines seems to promote slumber. Many night-workers, for instance, sleep much better for taking a light supper or a hot drink with a biscuit just before retiring. It is difficult to get to sleep on " an empty stomach," or at least when the stomach has been empty so long that gnawing and hunger are felt. On the other hand, an overloaded stomach is not conducive to refreshing sleep, although that condition makes one drowsy. In cases where indigestion produces insomnia no food should be taken four hours or more before sleeping time, or, if this is found to be disadvantageous, the food should be of the lightest description.

The prescription frequently made for chronic insomnia is that of rest or a vacation. Unfortunately both of these recommendations are usually more easily given than taken. Absolute vacancy of mind is talked about but never attained, and relief from mental activity means in reality relief from the habitual current of anxious thought, from care and responsibility, matters which in such cases are apt to be beyond the control of the physician. It is to be remembered that the disturbances of sleep which are the most difficult to manage come from within; and if a vacation is taken the occupation must be such as will displace morbid activities by healthy ones, not intense, but sufficient to predominate. If the patient has nothing else to think about, he will be sure to think of his troubles.

The most dangerous of all counterfeits of sleep is that induced by drugs. At the present day, when so many, either from choice or necessity, spend their time in passing from one form of excitement to another, when such an enormous amount of work or play has to be got through in a limited number of hours, it is not to be wondered at that sleeplessness is so common a trouble, or that specifics for its relief should be so eagerly sought after and so recklessly employed. It goes without saying that there is no drug that can produce physiological sleep; there are many which produce a state of unconsciousness resembling sleep, and some of these are unfortunately much resorted to for this purpose. Though permissible in skilled hands their habitual use is dangerous, both because they are all poisons and because they smother the symptom, suppress a danger signal, without doing anything to relieve the diseased condition which causes it. The man who works all day in an ill-ventilated room and takes little or no exercise, or the woman who slaves over her housework or her needlework or embroidery and almost forgets that there is such a thing as open air, the business man who is driving himself too hard and keeps up on stimulants, the individual who is in the early stage of some disease, when they find that they cannot sleep, instead of regarding it as nature's danger signal, demanding investigation and change of habits, swallow some sleeping draught and persist in their suicidal course until a breakdown results, that they can no longer shut their eyes to. There is no such thing as uncaused sleeplessness any more than there is uncaused loss of appetite, of strength, or weight. All of them are signals of trouble and should be promptly regarded and investigated as such. Narcotics have their place in medicine like other poisonous drugs, but that place is becoming steadily smaller as cases are more painstakingly and intelligently studied.

The sense of well-being and illusory strength induced by alcohol and other stimulants, and the sleep so easily procured by drugs, are specially dangerous to the nervous person whose moral courage and self-control are at fault. He readily falls a victim to narcotic indulgence. The sleeplessness which is often so distressing and exhausting is frequently only an expression of the nervous irritability and obsessions of the sufferer. Temporarily to dull his sensibilities with drugs is a sure way of intensifying the condition which it should be our endeavour to remedy in some more rational manner.

Of course, no doctor will forget that sleeplessness is frequently a symptom of bodily trouble, and that it is necessary to discover the underlying cause. We may have to remedy digestive derangements, to relieve local irritations, to correct disturbances of circulation, to relieve anæmia and debilitated conditions, and to secure due regard to sanitary requirements.

A large number of cases, especially those suffering from insomnia through worry, anxiety, overwork, and other mental conditions, can be cured by "suggestion," and this method is often effective even when organic causes are the trouble. Thus it has been my good fortune to send to sleep almost instantaneously a patient suffering from cancer, who was kept awake by pain for which morphia injections had ceased to give relief.

Obstinate cases often do well by the application of mild currents of electricity, especially galvanism. Its value is not sufficiently recognised. In happy contrast to the influence of sleep-compelling drugs, which are frequently a source of danger and usually occasion unpleasant sensations on the day following their administration, electricity, when administered carefully by a qualified medical man, induces a sleep that is pleasant in character and has no evil consequences. Further, not only is sleep produced, but the patient derives general benefit from the influence of electric currents. Sometimes the result is immediate, at other times a more prolonged course of treatment is required. I have found the effects to be not merely temporary, but permanent.

Often a combination of electrical treatment

and psychotherapeutics achieves the desired end. Anyhow, in the great majority of cases sleep can be procured without the aid of drugs, and astonishing successes are not infrequent even after powerful drugs have failed.

CHAPTER V

NERVOUS DYSPEPSIA

THE great majority of the dyspeptics of the present day are so because their nervous power has run down, or has been incontinently consumed in other directions without any regard for the needs of the stomach. It is positively rare to observe cases of nervous disorders without digestive troubles. They vary infinitely as to intensity and symptomatology. In some cases indigestion is the principal symptom complained of, and the mistake is made by the inexperienced and unqualified of treating by local measures indigestion which originates in a disordered nervous system.

In health there is a blessed unconsciousness of the very existence of a stomach; but if dyspepsia be present the patient can think of little else. A healthy man does not know that he has such a thing as a stomach, a dyspeptic does not know that he has anything else. With the neurotic, the dyspepsia is an abiding trouble;

he is obsessed by his gastric symptoms, dwells upon them continually, sits in judgment upon every article of food presented to him, yet it is obvious to everyone that if it were not the stomach it would be some other organ that would be occupying his thoughts.

Once certain people get the notion that they are troubled with indigestion, their minds dwell on it to such an extent that they are likely to limit their eating more than they should, and to disturb digestive processes by thinking about them, and using up in worry nervous energy that should be allowed to flow down to actuate digestion.

Nervous patients often say they have no appetite, that even though they eat, their food has no taste. Such people have lost their eating instinct to a certain degree. They eat merely from routine, or because food is placed before them. They would usually just as soon not eat. If a number of courses are presented to them, they eat such as they care for and take a conventional amount of each kind of food presented, but they have no particular feeling to guide them in the matter of quantity.

Dyspepsia is probably much more dependent on the mental state than on any other factor. At moments of depression, just after bad news has been received, the appetite is absent, or is very slight, and digestion itself proceeds slowly and unsatisfactorily. On the other hand, when there is a cheerful mental condition, appetite is vigorous and digestion is usually quite capable of disposing of all that is eaten. The unfavourable influence of the mind on digestion is seen in all those who are particular about their food. Everyone knows how repulsive may be the feeling produced by being told that something eaten with a relish contained some unusual ingredient, or was cooked under unclean conditions. Food that agrees quite well with people, so long as they do not know too much about it, often fails to be beneficial after they have seen how it has been prepared.

Sedentary occupations, involving mental work and little physical effort, seem especially to predispose to some form of indigestion. Few of those who live what is called the intellectual life escape suffering from some of its symptoms. In many cases dyspepsia is primarily due to over-concentration of attention on digestion. In others it is due to over-occupation with business, worry, or serious thought, at times when the digestive processes need all the energy. Men are at work from 10 to 6, and often enough bring home their professional or business worries with them, their brains being all the while in a state of turmoil. In the midst of this they eat and drink, and expect their stomachs to digest. But if they have exhausted their nervous supplies, where is the stomach to get its motive power ? The tired man, even though he may be hungry, can only eat a hearty meal at the risk of serious disturbance of digestion. In these days of hurry-scurry, our brains run ahead and take no thought for the stomach, and in consequence there is almost a necessity for many of us to suffer from a slow digestion. And a slow digestion means that as regards symptoms there will be more or less distension after food.

The habit of indulging in excessive meals is another cause of dyspepsia. The patient is often a highly-strung and vigorous person, who exhausts himself by his work, and feels stimulated and sustained by food, and eats more than he can digest, though he may obtain temporary relief by eating. Or he is very fond of the pleasures of the table, and having a good appetite, between his attacks he is led to indulge it whenever any dish to which he is especially partial is before him. Many of these people are not aware that they are eating more than is good for them, for the ordinary estimate of the

necessary amount is far too high. Overfeeding
leads to flatulence, drowsiness, and a loss of the
wonted energy. The fortunes of the quack pill
vendors show the extent of this vice. Every
man should rise from table not satiated, but
wishing to eat more.

Very few men realise also the fact that the
process of digestion uses up nervous power.
Most people imagine that the more they eat the
more strength they will acquire; whereas the
truth is that beyond the amount of food needed
by each individual to repair waste in proportion
to his expenditure in muscular or mental work,
the rest is superfluous, and consumes in the
disposal of it nervous energy that might otherwise be utilised in more valuable ways.

The gastric symptoms due to failure of nervous
power are characterised by their extreme
irregularity, the patient not uncommonly feeling
very ill one day and quite well the next without
obvious reason for the change. The most
constant complaint is of vague discomfort,
which rarely amounts to actual pain. It is
generally worst in the morning and decreases
toward evening; it is increased after meals, a
sensation of fullness being felt as soon as a small
quantity has been eaten.

The discomfort has little relation to the

amount or the kind of food taken ; it is increased by worry and excitement, whilst some new interest, whether it be a change of surroundings, the visit of a friend, or a new medicine, leads to its temporary disappearance. Thus, when alone or with dull company, food of any kind may be simply repulsive, and, if taken, may induce a painful sensation. But the same food, taken in the company of congenial associates, may be not only enjoyed by the palate, but digested with ease and comfort. Often the patients feel worse when the stomach is empty and are relieved by eating. In others the symptoms come on after eating, though, perhaps, not until several hours have elapsed. The appetite is always diminished, especially when there is worry or anxiety, though it varies considerably from day to day. As insufficient food is taken the nervous system becomes more depressed ; this reacts again on the digestion, a vicious circle being produced. Most patients complain of flatulence, which may be nothing more than the result of misinterpreting the sensation of fullness, no excess of gas being present. Nausea sometimes occurs, and occasionally vomiting.

These patients are almost always irritable and find difficulty in exercising sufficient self-control to make life pleasant to themselves and their friends. We know very well how our feelings vary with our bodily condition, how dismal the world looks during a fit of indigestion, and what a host of evils disappear as the abused stomach regains its tone. The effect of indigestion may be seen in the records of history and literature. It has led to the loss of battles ; it has caused many crimes and inspired much sulphurous theology, gloomy poetry, and bitter satire.

On the other hand, the influence of the brain on digestion has not escaped the observation of physicians in any age. The effects of the emotions—such as love, anger, worry, and anxiety—on the appetite are found described in the literature of the ancients.

Seeing what important influence the mental and nervous states have upon digestion, we must not be misled into treating the purely local symptoms as quacks do, judging by their eloquent advertisements in the daily Press; but once having assured ourselves by a thorough examination that there is no organic cause for the trouble complained of by the patient, we must study him as a whole, not only from the point of view of his animal functions but from the psychological point of view. We must consider not only what he eats or drinks, but be interested in what he thinks.

There is hardly a patient suffering from nervous dyspepsia who has not tried one or more quack nostrums. Much mischief is done in this way. What these patients do not know is that their indigestion is merely a symptom and not the disease they are suffering from. On the other hand, until they have been examined by a physician they cannot know whether this indigestion is, or is not, a sign of organic and maybe even malignant disease.

The proper treatment is to study first of all the causation of the disorder, and to do this a perfectly clear diagnosis is necessary. A patient may come complaining simply of indigestion, when a careful and tactful examination will reveal the cause in the shape of some depressing circumstance. In such a case neither drugs nor diet, but a change in some life circumstance, gives the clue to successful treatment. If the indigestion is due merely to nervous exhaustion, we must raise the nervous power ; we must remember that the indigestion is not the disease, and that we have to treat the patient's main disorder—his nervous debility.

Only after we have corrected all extraneous sources of trouble should we attend to the diet. This is just the opposite rule from that which obtains amongst this class of dyspeptics. They are too fond of " pampering " the stomach. A man who continuously and anxiously considers the kind of food he eats—whether it is going to agree with him or not when he eats it—is a dyspeptic, and will always remain so. The vast majority of men are led by their instincts to a reasonably nutritious and sensible dietary, and the more completely we can keep our minds off our digestions and the " chemical " choice of our food, the better it is for us. The individual who thinks the world is going to be saved by eating brown bread or any other article of diet, regardless of the fact that what agrees with one may upset another, is a crank. It is not even well for us to consider too nicely the amount of water or food taken, or whether it is digestible or not. The really healthy stomach ought to be and is capable of disposing of not only the digestible and the difficult of digestion, but the indigestible. Any other kind of stomach is not worth having.

What is the use to the invalid patient to be told of the nutritive properties of certain foods, when he never assimilates them. We must prescribe foods which the particular stomach will digest. All cases of nervous disorder want guidance and moral influence, more particularly in reference to diet than to any other curative agent; and each stomach must be treated according to its own respective requirements, and, I might even go so far as to say, its own peculiarities. A patient should be guided largely by his own experience of what is good and bad for him. We must not forget that some perfectly wholesome foods are literal poisons to certain stomachs, and those which after repeated trials steadily disagree had better be avoided. If prejudice exists with regard to certain foods, there will be no relish for them; and unless these prejudices can be removed the foods either will not be taken, though they represent important nutritional elements, or else they will be taken in such small quantities and digested with so much consciousness of their presence and such difficulty as to be a disturbing factor for health.

For food to be digested, it must first of all be attractive to the taste. If it be unattractive it will not stimulate the juices indispensable to good digestion. Without appetite there can be no healthy digestion, and foods that pall on the appetite are just as surely defective as foods as those that are deficient in nutritive value. The dyspeptic who is confident that a certain food will disagree with him is almost sure to experience indigestion if he eats that particular food.

Many persons of middle age suffer through a monotony of diet. Our aims should be to keep our food range as wide as possible. Anything which tends to limit and monotonise diet exercises an injurious effect upon the general vigour of the system. Both stomach and bowels may be trained to perform their work regularly. Habit means probably more with these organs than any other factor. Our digestive tract is largely dependent on habit. We get hungry three times a day or twice a day, according to the custom that we have established. Countries differ radically in the matter; and nearly always, when a man goes from one country to another in early years, he changes to the habits of the new country, though if he goes after middle age he usually clings to those that he is used to.

If we accustom ourselves to dining every day at a particular hour, every day at that hour the stomach will become congested and secrete gastric juice without any intervention of our will. If, for once, we give it nothing to eat, it will suffer and cry famine ; if for a long time together we disturb its habits, and the hours of our meals become irregular, the stomach gets out of order.

If, to digest our food, we should enjoy it, it should of course be taken leisurely and in a pleasant frame of mind. The cheerful society of friends should not be absent; and the longer time spent over the meal enjoyed in company, the greater the benefit from it. Next to anxiety, the worst foe to digestion is hurry. Haste cuts short mastication, and on the perfection of that process chiefly depends the rapidity with which the assimilation of the food can be effected. The actual indication of a sufficiency of food is the feeling of satisfaction, not satiety, which is always a symptom of excess. This feeling of perfect comfort the hurried eater cannot know.

The patient should not be too fatigued before commencing a meal, otherwise the stomach will not work efficiently. If he is too tired a few minutes' mental as well as physical rest should be allowed. Rest from work is again advisable after the meal, to give the stomach an opportunity of placing its machinery in running order. Many people immediately after a meal jump up from the table, continue whatever business or pleasure is in hand, and never give a thought to the long-suffering and patient stomach, until the stomach gives its owner some discomfort or pain. The hours at which meals are taken, then, must be so arranged as to avoid the system being tired when it tackles the food ; and to allow of a little rest after the meal to start the complicated process of digestion freely on its way.

The quantity of food required to keep one in sound condition varies so largely that it is impossible to lay down more than a tentative average standard. The quality is a matter of custom and environment; here, too, no rigid universal rule can be enforced. Doubtless, most of us eat too much. Vegetarianism suits some, but for the bulk of mankind mixed diet is the best.

Quite a number of people take too much salt with their food, and in this way aggravate the tendency to acidity; others are too fond of highly seasoned food or of pastry or sweet things; or, again, the quantity of liquid imbibed at a meal may be too large. In such cases a careful revision of the diet is absolutely necessary.

Often a change of environment that takes patients away from the ordinary cares of life is sufficient to make all the difference between ease of digestion and extremely uncomfortable dyspepsia.

It is evident from what has been said that it is extremely unwise for patients to treat themselves and still more foolish to indulge in quack remedies. It is only a qualified physician who can judge whether the indigestion is a symptom of organic or functional disorder, and whether it is due to local disturbance or is a sign of debility of the nervous system in general.

Nervous dyspepsia is another of those disorders which are most amenable to " suggestion." I have seen even chronic vomiting relieved by it. After all, it is nothing more wonderful than the fact known to seafaring men that those who direct a ship cease to be seasick when its safety is in danger. At the same time, while insisting on the importance of the mind in the treatment of these functional disorders of digestion, this does not imply that tonic remedies which stimulate the appetite and add tone to the muscles of the stomach should not be used when duly indicated. They are often helpful. If prescribed in connection with changes in the patient's habits, and especially such as direct his attention away from his digestive tract, and from wrong persuasions as to food-taking, the good they accomplish will be lasting.

Let me add a few words about CONSTIPATION. There are more people sick because of it than for any other reason. Any number of special causes may be at the root of constipation, but the commonest is certainly physical inactivity. Another cause lies in the kind of food we eat. We take so much trouble nowadays to have it nourishing, digestible and perfectly prepared, that we often fail to give the stomach and intestines enough work to do. " Predigested " and " concentrated " foods have a place in the world, but it is not that of a regular diet.

Another sure method of achieving constipation is that of delaying to answer the calls of the system when they come. If a man kept a regular time each day for attending to the business of disposing of the waste products of his body, the system would soon adjust itself and be ready to respond at the right moment. Regularity in this matter is essential to healthy living.

Often enough, the root of the difficulty lies not so much in bad habits of the body as in bad habits of mind. Worry and nervousness weaken the digestion. Discouragement and low spirits lead the straight road to constipation. Melancholy tends to aid constipation and constipation tends towards melancholy.

Then there is the practice of using laxatives. It lies at the back of thousands of chronic cases of constipation. A man who uses a laxative to help him out of an inconvenience is not hitting at the root of the difficulty at all. The conditions that gave rise to it will probably remain, and they will make trouble again.

CHAPTER VI

NERVOUS DISORDERS OF THE HEART, CIRCULATION, AND RESPIRATION

THE heart has its own special work to do, and will do it well if left alone, but it constitutes a centre to receive and to distribute sympathy, through its nervous connections, greater than that of any other organ in the body. Everyone is only too familiar with the way in which the heart becomes affected by anything which disturbs the feelings, the emotions, and the receptive nerve centres. The action of the heart is most natural and regular when it is least thought of. On the other hand, emotional disturbances act unfavourably upon the heart and blood vessels. Any agitation of the mind almost immediately produces a conscious thumping of the heart against the chest wall. Worry, suspense, anxious anticipation, disappointment, consciousness of failure or of failing health, the " hunted " feeling that comes of overwork and arrears, regret, sorrow, despair—all such depressing influences wear out not only the nervous system, with which they are immediately related, but the cardio-vascular system as well.

The nervous heart presents three typical characteristic features, which are exemplified by the rapidity, the tension, and the irregularity of the pulse. Excitability of the pulse is a common feature. The least thing—any little noise, the presence of a stranger, or any slight excitement —will start the pulse off at a very rapid and often irregular rate. The pulsations of the heart are distinctly felt by the patient as palpitations and are attended with more or less severe pain in the region of the apex. In some cases, however, there is no real disturbance, but that in some way the heart action has become noticeable to the patient.

Palpitation is a condition in which one is conscious of the beating of the heart; the severity varies from a mere sensation of fluttering to a violent and tumultuous throbbing and hammering of the heart against the chest wall, causing acute distress. These palpitations, and the distressing sensations by which they are accompanied, disturb the minds of the patients, who soon believe themselves to be affected with some grave lesion of the heart. As a matter of fact, these attacks have no gravity, but they return frequently, and their reappearance occurs under the influence of the most diverse and often the most trifling causes ; a slight emotion, even a moderate physical effort, or the work of digestion, suffices to provoke them.

Often the beginning of the cardiac unrest is found in some stomachic symptoms. The distension of the stomach with gas is often a mechanical reason for interference with the heart action. The patient complains of heart trouble when he is really suffering from indigestion.

The excessive smoker, especially the cigarette smoker, often complains of palpitation of the heart. He complains that this palpitation wakens him in the middle of the night, when he finds that his heart is beating violently, and that he feels restless and uncomfortable, and that he cannot go to sleep again until the heart has quietened down.

In the nervous heart caused by worry and anxiety, the heart is so irritable, so ill-tempered, so fractious, and so sensitive that it—figuratively speaking—tumbles about, kicks, starts, and plunges in a manner which becomes exceedingly distressing and almost unbearable. At times the slightest movement of the body will produce this effect, walking upstairs, ascending a hill, reading an article which touches the feelings, or eating or drinking anything which disagrees.

H

The heart, like the brain, is a creature of habit. If it once gets out of training and assumes vicious propensities it takes a vast deal of moral persuasion, and something more, to put it right again.

To give useful advice to a man whose heart and vessels present evidences of wearing out from nervous stress is not an easy task. The physician or practitioner who undertakes this responsible duty should possess not only professional knowledge, based on experience, but an intimate acquaintance with the affairs of life, and as far as possible an insight into the character, disposition and circumstances, personal, domestic and public, of the individual.

Medicines in such cases are seldom of use. If there are some cases where they act favourably by suggestion, there are others, more numerous, where the use of an anodyne gives to the disease the stamp of reality, which is exactly what it ought not to have in the patient's mind. It awakens the idea of an organic affection when the first consideration of the physician ought to be to dissipate all fear and all idea of danger. Many functional disturbances of the heart will disappear entirely with judicious regulation of life, hygienic living and psychotherapy. The removal of inhibiting influences originating in the mind and the suggestion of favourable mental influences are as important for the heart as for the other organs of the body.

Whilst it is not always necessary, and frequently is highly inadvisable, to stop work altogether, there must be a limit to the amount and length of even purely intellectual work, and sufficient provision must be made for sleep, recreation, and distraction. The patient must be freed from worry, which is often very difficult, and he must beware of mental occupation of a nature which at an unexpected moment may provoke emotional excitement in the form of vexation or passion. The most important condition of all is that the patient does not worry over his condition, for that hampers his heart's action still further.

Patients suffering from these functional derangements of the heart often make them a pretext for avoiding exercise and for taking stimulants, whereas exercise and fresh air are what they need. Exercise of some kind or another is one of the important features of all the health resorts which specialise in the treatment of heart diseases, and as it has to be arranged according to the individual condition, the patient should not neglect to consult a properly qualified physician.

Sometimes the nervous attack of the heart leads to a sensation of GIDDINESS, when the patient feels like fainting. Surrounding objects appear clouded and swaying and the patient is in need of steadying himself by holding on to something. Giddiness may arise from other causes and a correct diagnosis is of first importance for successful treatment.

In other cases there are attacks of nervous palpitation and great discomfort about the heart, resembling ANGINA PECTORIS, which is a serious affection, and also common in nervous sufferers. It is frequently a source of terror and anxiety for the persons attacked by it, and is peculiarly apt to throw them into a state of extreme dejection and depression.

The pseudo-angina may resemble a true attack. The patient suddenly experiences in the region of the heart a feeling as of being gripped, a sensation of constriction, which quickly becomes extremely painful and radiates immediately into the left shoulder and arm. He is a prey to anguish, to inexpressible terror. His breathing is short and quick; his face pale and livid; his extremities are pale, cold, and apparently bloodless. The pulse is small and feeble, and the heart-beats are almost imperceptible. After a duration of some minutes the crisis terminates

by an evident change in the state of the circulation.   The face becomes red and hot ;   the
energy of the heart-beats increases, and everything returns into order.   Emotional excitement
and mental anxiety figure very largely in the
formation of pseudo-angina.

True angina occurs in most cases in consequence
of hardening of the arteries of the heart or of
some valvular lesion that interferes in some way
with cardiac nutrition.   A definite sign is arterial
degeneration in various parts of the body.   When
there are no signs of arterial degeneration and no
significant murmurs in the heart, it should be
made clear to these patients that they are not
suffering from a fatal disease, but only from a
bothersome nervous manifestation, which is
compatible not only with continued good health
but with long life.   It must not be forgotten
that neurotic patients exaggerate their pains and
describe their distress in the heart region as
extremely severe, when all they mean is that,
because their pain is near their heart, it produces
an extreme solicitude and that a dread of death
comes over them because of this anxiety.   For
the treatment of pseudo-angina, mental influence
is all-important.

Besides the nervous heart, there are numerous
DISORDERS OF THE CIRCULATION.   From the

sympathetic system of nerves come tiny nerve twigs which lie along the blood vessels and regulate the circulation in the various parts of the body and limbs. When these little automatic regulators are weak and irritable they render the patient over-susceptible not only to external conditions, such as atmospheric changes, causing chills, pallor, " dead fingers " sensation, etc., but to internal conditions, as produced by the various emotions, which then cause *blushing, flushing,* and *abnormal perspiration.*

MORBID BLUSHING although not, strictly speaking, a serious disorder, is, to say the least, extremely disagreeable to the victim. It is simply the manifestation of a weakness in the nervous system. Probably the most prominent exciting cause is self-consciousness, either by introspection or by the attention being drawn to the external portions of the body while under examination by others. If a modest individual of a delicate nervous organisation is in company with a number of persons, and imagines that the people around him are regarding him critically and are entertaining rather a disparaging opinion of him, he is very liable to manifest his abnormal self-consciousness by blushing, or even by becoming embarrassed in his conversation, and stammering. Blushing is common in those of delicate nervous organisation, while those of coarse natures are very little affected by it. Many cultivated and scientific men are prone to blush inordinately from humility and diffidence, having a low opinion of their own ability, while the ignorant egotist is never known to blush. Blushing rarely occurs in solitude or in darkness ; it occurs most often when observation is directed towards the personal appearance, and then results from embarrassment and self-consciousness. Many of these inordinate blushers are timid and melancholic. They seek solitude and are excessively sensitive when meeting people. Many of the victims of this disorder, if relating an incident or anecdote, will often lose the thread of the story by their concern as to what their auditors may be thinking of them.

In severe cases the mental confusion is very marked, the heart throbs violently, there is a sensation of suffocation, and the breath becomes short. There is a peculiar sensation at the pit of the stomach often followed by constriction of the throat. Palpitation of the heart is a very common condition immediately preceding the act of blushing. Many blushers experience a feeling of dread as part of the emotional state.

In a large number of cases the individual completely loses the power of thought for the time being. The mind is completely paralysed, and, in popular language, he is "covered with confusion." There is an instinctive desire for self-concealment. The blusher either averts the head or looks downward. The expression, "I wished I could have sunk through the floor," which is sometimes used, aptly expresses the mental condition of the patient at this time. When a person has once suffered from this disorder, he is liable to have subsequent attacks; for the nervous system is highly impressionable, and the condition once well developed is apt to be perpetuated by slight influence.

Blushing is generally confined to the face on account of its extreme vascularity, and therefore having a great supply of vasomotor nerves; the face, moreover, being the portion of the body most exposed to view and upon which attention is concentrated in looking for recognition, or in studying character or discerning beauty or homeliness.

For purposes of treatment one must go back to the origin of the mental trouble and dispel the primary morbid mental condition, the self-consciousness, uneasiness, shyness, timidity, and the various preoccupations which drive the blood to the face, and one must give the patient confidence in himself.

Here we must discuss also NERVOUS DISORDERS. OF RESPIRATION. One often notices disturbances of the respiration in nervous patients; slight acceleration of the respiratory movement, irregularities of rhythm, and sighs. Many complain of a purely subjective sensation of distress. Shortness of breath is often a harassing symptom. Much can be done for it by deliberate training in deep breathing and proper exercise.

ASTHMA, i.e. spasm of the bronchial tubes, is common in nervous patients. It may occur under many circumstances and is frequently secondary to some other disease; but true spasmodic asthma afflicts chiefly those of a nervous temperament and is brought on by emotional influences. It does not end fatally; but, when once contracted, exhibits a recurrent persistence which makes the sufferer's life miserable and drives him to one quack remedy after another, then to one doctor after another. It is certainly amenable to suggestion treatment by the elimination of the exciting causes and the ever-present psychical factor.

CHAPTER VII

HEADACHE, NEURALGIA, AND OTHER PAINS

HEADACHE is unquestionably the most common of all common ailments. In spite of the improvement in the general health of the community, due to more hygienic living, more healthy food and better ventilation, headache, instead of decreasing, has increased to a great degree. Any number of headache cures are advertised in the daily papers, in the street cars, on the signboards, even in medical journals, and besides these nearly every druggist has his own special preparation for headache, so it would seem as though literally many millions of doses of these headache cures must be taken every week.

There are, of course, organic headaches due to definite pathological conditions, but the great majority of headaches are the result of over-attention to certain sensations and queer feelings about the head, some of them normal, some of them only slightly abnormal, which are annoyances rather than pain and are emphasised by the concentration of attention on them until they become a torment. With regard to all headaches, even the most genuine variety, there are certain considerations that are of value. Most people think that it is the brain itself that is suffering pain, and not a little of their suffering is due to the fact that they dread the effect of such pain upon the brain tissues and its possible consequences upon their mental state. Such people will be much relieved to be told at once that the brain itself is not sensitive, has no feeling, and when exposed it may be touched with impunity without causing any pain. It is the structures surrounding the brain that are sensitive. It is not the pressure upon the brain tissue itself that is the underlying cause of the pain, but pressure upon the sensitive structures connected with the brain. Patients find their pain much more bearable as soon as they are assured that headaches do not lead to mental disturbances.

The symptoms vary somewhat when it is purely a nervous headache and when a nervous headache is associated with an anæmic, hyperæmic, or toxic condition of the blood.

Nervous headache is a dull, nagging ache together with a sense of pressure. In certain cases there is a constant feeling as though the head were weighted down by a heavy helmet, or as though it were itself too heavy for the shoulders and tended to fall backward. Oftentimes there is a sensation of burning in the scalp, and the area involved actually feels hot to the touch. Many other annoying sensations in this region are also complained of, notably a feeling as if the scalp were drawn tightly over the skull or as if it were encompassed by a constricting band. The most familiar sensations referred to the interior of the skull are those of fullness or emptiness, lightness or heaviness. Practically all these uncomfortable feelings, whether they appear to emanate from the scalp or from within the skull, are increased by mental application.

The proximate cause of *anœmic headache* is deficiency of blood within the cranial cavity. It is a common sequence of all forms of debility. Sometimes those affected by this variety of headache complain of a sensation of tightness about the forehead ; sometimes the pain manifests itself in clawing sensations, which are particularly well marked at the vertex. Whatever the location of the pain may be, it is almost invariably less pronounced when the subject is in the recumbent position than when the body is maintained in an erect attitude. Less pain is therefore felt during the latter part of the night and early morning than during the day. In the more serious cases the simple act of rising is sufficient to cause vertigo and even fainting ; indeed symptoms of giddiness and weakness in the lower extremities are almost constant accompaniments of this form of headache.

In hyperæmic and congestive headache the subject complains of a severe tensive pain, and at the same time experiences a sensation of fullness, as though the cranium were too small for its contents. As a rule the painful sensations are not circumscribed in character, but are distributed throughout the entire extent of the cranium. The pain is constant, and is augmented by assuming the recumbent posture ; consequently sleep is more or less profoundly affected. All forms of mental or physical exertion are followed by exacerbations of pain accompanied by more or less giddiness. Sensory disturbances are also common, and may consist in functional exaltation or depression. The subject is extremely irritable and may be aroused to inordinate passion by the most trivial circumstances ; he is pessimistic, depressed, and lachrymose, and inclined to find fault with all about him.

Toxic headache is caused by some chemical change in the constitution of the blood. Sometimes the subject complains of a heavy, dull sensation in the head, which may or may not be accompanied by giddiness. Again, the pain is sharp, and is described as splitting or boring. According to the extent of the intoxication, the faculties of the mind are more or less affected. There may be actual delirium as in violent febrile disturbances, or the only symptoms noticed may be heaviness and slight mental confusion.

Migraine, sick or bilious headache, comes on in paroxysms and is frequently one-sided. Fatigue and excitement, digestive disturbance, and over-stimulation of the eyes are likely to bring on an attack, which is generally accompanied by nausea and vomiting.

For the treatment of headache I have rarely had to employ drugs in all my varied experience. A headache powder does not grapple with the cause of the headache any more than a laxative affects the cause of constipation or a spoonful of pepsin the cause of indigestion. We have cut out the symptoms, but the root of the trouble is still untouched. In headache, as in other ailments, our first duty is to ascertain the cause. By removal of the cause we can get rid of the symptom. Having eliminated any organic source of irritation, such as eye-strain, for example, and attended to the constitutional requirements, we must correct any hygienic transgression and faulty mental attitude by psychotherapy, to which we shall refer in greater detail when we speak of pain further on in this chapter. When the headache is really severe I have frequently found the application of a weak galvanic current to the affected region most efficacious, the pain being removed almost instantaneously, probably owing to the influence of the electricity on the circulation and on the brain cells.

Frequently the patients complain not of headache but of NOISES IN THE HEAD, which are sometimes so loud and continuous as to become most disturbing. We exclude, of course, those noises due to ear disease. We are dealing only with such causes as variations in the quantity, quality, and pressure of the blood, either in the ear itself or in the brain, such as are induced in adults by worry, excitement, fatigue, debility, or indigestion. These noises may be either ringing, whistling, hissing, cracking, pulsating, soft blowing, continuous or intermittent. In many cases all these sounds are absent, but the subject is still greatly annoyed by hearing the beat of his pulse in the ear when his head is on the pillow.

Nothing can be imagined more painful or harder to bear than a continual noise in the ears such as some unfortunate patients describe. The enjoyment of life is destroyed, the temper soured, and the power of work greatly reduced. It is exceptional that patients get accustomed to the noise in their ears, and are able to follow the advice so freely tendered to them by their doctors and friends, that they should forget all about it and think of something else ; on the contrary, in the large majority of cases no amusement or change of occupation and scene has the slightest influence upon it, and the trouble is felt as keenly after it has lasted for years as it was when it first began. Still, it is by " suggestion " treatment that the best results are achieved.

PAIN IN THE BACK AND LIMBS is not uncommon in nervous exhaustion. The spine may be tender to pressure. There may be disinclination to move or twist the body, but not so marked as in lumbago, sprain, or more serious and deeper troubles. It is very important that an accurate diagnosis should be made.

With these spinal pains there is often a general HYPERÆSTHESIA or OVER-SENSITIVENESS. The patient, not unfrequently, is painfully sensitive to heat and to cold, to a depressing atmosphere, and to every change of wind. Patients may be so sensitive that a slight draught or the slamming of a door gives rise to acute pain. " Numbness," " coldness," " deadness," and other sensations of the hands and feet are also common.

Hypersensitiveness is a common sign of fatigue. A noise that one does not hear when one is rested will be perfectly distracting when one is tired. Instead of making the nervous system a less responsive instrument, fatigue makes it more responsive; more responsive but less serviceable. For at the same time that irritability is increased, power is decreased. Irritability and weakness usually go together. A loss of self-control in small things, that is the symptom described in different terms; but another name for it is irritability.

At first it seems odd that this undue sensitiveness to slight stimuli should be so sure an effect of fatigue; but it means that the resistance-gates are down, and we become aware of sensations pouring in from all sides, slight sensations that ordinarily we do not notice because—by the laws of attention—they are quietly shut out from our consciousness. But when our attention is tired—no longer focussed, but scattered, all these slight nerve pricks attack us insistently, and we cannot neglect them. We have all seen

I

—and, alas, been an integral part of—some
audience that was trying to endure the last half-
hour of an unendurable speech.　Everybody
was shifting his position, crossing one leg over
the other and back again, moving the fingers,
playing with watch-charms or chains, yawning,
twitching, folding programmes, wiping eye-
glasses, twisting moustaches.　Those are all
fatigue signs.

Often there is both a physical and mental
hypersensitiveness, the patient being peculiarly
alive to all sorts of sources of annoyance.　The
ordinary impressions made during everyday life
upon the senses, which to the healthy individual
are pleasant or indifferent, or at any rate easily
tolerable, become obtrusive evils; while the well-
meant efforts of friends, often in the direction
of social entertainment and amusement, are so
many further sources of irritation.　If such
patients are asked whether they are nervous
they are often indignant at the question, though
they readily own that they abhor the slightest
noise, or a domestic upset, and that they are
oversensitive to emotional stimuli.　Temper may
not be easily ruffled, but they are ready " to
jump out of their skin " at the jarring of a door,
and are in agony at hearing the leaves of a
book turned over.　To many the mere thought

of a saw being ground or of a pencil squeaking
on a slate, or of a cork being cut by a blunt
knife, produces a momentary shiver, goose-skin,
and a more or less lasting sense of discomfort.
It is torture to some to hear others converse ;
others say, that on the most trivial occurrence,
they " feel all of a tremble, all of a shake."

NEURALGIA, a painful condition of one or
more nerves, is also common. Such a neuralgic
attack is always preceded by a condition of
debility resulting from general or special causes.
The onset of the malady is usually heralded by
vague muscular twitchings or sensations of
pricking, quickly succeeded by evanescent dart-
ing pains. The pains are recurrent in character
and succeed each other with ever-increasing
frequency and intensity, until, in the more
severe attacks, the patient suffers the most
excruciating agony. These pains are sometimes
regional and are ascribed by the subject to
particular areas, which are found to correspond
to the course of a nerve trunk. At other times
they are ambulatory and dart from place to
place. The most common of the regional forms
are facial neuralgia and sciatica. Both these
affections are readily influenced by the application of galvanism to the affected nerve. Such,
at all events, is my personal experience. Of late,

since the introduction of radium, radium ionisation has given splendid results even in chronic cases, where the pain could previously be mitigated only by opium or morphia.

With reference to all these conditions of hypersensitiveness and pain, whether general or localised, physical or mental, psychotherapy is very important. For we must remember that the conditions are often due to such concentration of mind on a particular portion of the body that the ordinary sensations of that part, usually experienced quite unconsciously, become first a source of uneasy discomfort, and later an ache or pain. There may be some slight physical disturbance which calls attention to the part, but there is no really serious pathological condition. While such pains are spoken of as imaginary, it must be remembered that this does not mean that they are non-existent. On the contrary, they may be much more real to the patient than physical ailments. While pain may be thus created by concentration of attention, it must not be forgotten that what the mind can do in increasing pain is even more formidable than in originating it. Many a chronic pain is made worse by complaining about it and resisting it. If the pain were calmly accepted as a matter of fact, it would immediately lose much of its torturing power. It is the dread of pain which tempts so many patients to the use of drugs, which do serious harm, and for which a habit is easily acquired.

In functional disorders more than in any other we have to distinguish between the actual symptoms and the interpretation which the patient inevitably places upon these symptoms. Undoubtedly, the actual pains and aches and discomforts, great as they are, which nervous people endure, cause a less appreciable amount of suffering than the meanings which they assume these aches and pains and discomforts to convey. On the other hand, we must remember that people do not get nervous for the "fun of the thing." It is a somewhat superficial view which is condensed in the undoubtedly clever saying, that some folk "enjoy poor health." If they enjoy it, it is not ill-health to them, no matter what it may appear to be to those about them. There is no enjoyment about real ill-health, whether it be physical or mental in origin ; it is a serious and depressing business. It is extremely important to grasp the fact that patients suffering from functional nervous disorders are really suffering acutely, sometimes more acutely than patients with gross organic nerve disease. Because their symptoms are largely of a subjective character, and appear to one who does not suffer them as trifling and unreal, these patients are sometimes given to understand that there is really nothing the matter with them, that their trouble is purely imaginary; with the effect that they are driven into the hands of quacks, who are only too glad to claim a cure where doctors are supposed to have failed.

The sufferer seems always able to bear the pain that is present, and it is only the cumulative effect of the pain that is past and the anticipation of the discomfort to come that make the pain unbearable. Nearly always it is much more the dread of what the pain may mean, and the lack of power to endure, which gradually develops as a consequence of suffering, that constitute the worst features of pain. There are many neurotic people whose susceptibility to pain has been so much increased by their lack of self-control and their tendency to react easily to pain, that even slight pain becomes a torment. Habits of introspection and the lack of serious occupation of mind of many people leave them the victims of over-attention to themselves. The whole question of the treatment of pain involves the study of the individual much more than it does the affliction which causes the pain.

What seems unbearable pain to many may be little more than a passing annoyance to others. What would be, under ordinary circumstances, intolerable torture, especially to sensitive people, may, because of intense preoccupation of mind, remain absolutely unnoticed. For example, in the excitement of a panic men suffer what would, under other circumstances, be excruciating agony and yet do not know that they are hurt. The oversensitive patient must be trained to bear discomfort for a while until his mind is diverted to other things than the concentration of attention on those functions which is causing their disturbance.

CHAPTER VIII

LOSS OF MUSCULAR CONTROL

NERVOUS TREMORS AND MUSCULAR SPASMS

As before stated, a tired feeling is often the first symptom of nervous exhaustion. The first sign is usually a feeling of undue muscular weariness after moderate or even slight exertion, such as a short walk. The patient finds that his legs soon get tired, and by degrees he becomes conscious of the fact that exercise is no longer a source of enjoyment. The sufferer rises more or less exhausted in the morning, and his exhaustion tends to increase until late in the afternoon, when, curiously enough, he usually begins to improve. Any form of activity which involves the co-ordinated use of certain muscles quickly brings on a feeling of exhaustion in these muscles.

As the exhaustion becomes more or less chronic other symptoms arise, such as MUSCULAR RESTLESSNESS AND UNCERTAINTY OF THEIR ACTION. Indeed, the world seems filled with nervous, fidgety persons, who are constantly engaged in numerous physical activities which are wholly useless and unnecessary. Among such nervous activities are wriggling movements of the body, inability to hold the hands naturally and composedly, resulting in restless movements of them; restless movements of the fingers, twiddling of an object, such as a pencil, biting the nails, general tremor, bending of the legs, inco-ordinate gait; or, if sitting, fidgeting of the legs, crossing and recrossing them, tossing the foot, tapping the foot on the floor, beating an incessant tattoo with the hands on the chair Some part of their anatomy must be in rhythmical and incessant action. Others will twist their moustaches or play with the hair. Others are everlastingly fixing their clothes or adjusting their necktie; they seem never to be able to complete their toilet. Some are addicted to giggling, to "nervous laughter," "sheepish" expression, or inability to look one straight in the face, the eyes glancing up, down, on one side, or askance, and these physical signs are accompanied often by mental confusion, flurry, the employment of wrong words, the making of ridiculous remarks and the doing of ridiculous things.

These unconscious muscular actions, habitual gestures and tricks of physiognomy are more or less distinctive of classes. There is the rustic who scratches his head, the horseman who whips his riding-boot, the thinker who finds inspiration in fingering his beard or tearing paper to pieces, the heavy dragoon who tugs at his moustache, the old drum-major who twirls his cane, the bashful girl who puts a finger in her mouth or who bites her nails, the impatient visitor who is kept waiting and drums with his fingers on window-panes or tables, and persons who whilst talking nervously move their legs.

All these needless and useless actions constitute a tremendous nervous and vital drain on the victim's constitution, a constant leakage of nervous force and muscular energy.

Such patients should exercise persistent quiet discipline ; but when they are told of this and are persuaded to attempt it they make such determined effort to overcome the affection that they make themselves more conscious of it than before, with the result that their movements are emphasised. Therefore we have to teach the patient how to relax both his mind and muscles by suggestion and auto-suggestion.

There is generally some amount of MUSCULAR TREMOR. Tremor is, of course, natural in certain conditions. Besides being an expression of weakness, as in old age, or fatigue, or the feebleness of convalescence, or of organic disease, or toxic states, tremor is a sign in many people of transient emotion, of fear, of excitement, of anger, or of grief; it is as natural a motor expression in some mobile natures as laughter or crying is of uncontrolled mirth or grief. Such tremor is capable in nervous persons of passing over the line of healthy functional manifestation and becoming a symptom of disorder and lack of emotional control.

Once a tremor has been observed by the nervous subject, a fear arises of trembling again, and this, together with the discomfort which it causes the subject who experiences it, increases the emotion which makes the trembling lasting. Tremors also persist by reason of the very state of contraction into which the subject puts himself when he becomes concerned about his tremors and tries to stop them. Hence in the treatment it is important to remove the " fear " of tremor, besides attending to the general health.

Some patients suffer from muscular spasms, so-called NERVOUS TICS, arising from emotional excitement, mental and physical shock, strain or exhaustion, and any condition which lowers the general health. A tic is a psychical affection in which the inhibitory power of the will is so feeble that a movement which originally served a definite purpose becomes exaggerated and can be controlled only, if at all, at the cost of great mental discomfort. The tiqueur realises the foolishness of his tic, and a conflict occurs between the illogical desire to perform it and the logical desire to restrain it.

In simple tics the facial muscles are most often affected, but the head, shoulders, or arms may also be involved, and sniffing or coughing and every variety of weird sound may also occur. Often it is originally merely a response to some irritation, as, for instance, when the eye is screwed up in the effort to see with an uncorrected error of refraction. This motor response is normal, but it becomes abnormal when it continues after its cause has disappeared, as it then no longer serves any useful purpose. An occasional blink is thus replaced by a series of futile flickerings of the eyelids. It is seldom that more than one tic is practised at a time. Some special kind of grimace may persist for days or weeks and then cease as suddenly as it began, only to give place to other forms of tic in succession. The tic becomes most evident upon excitement or fatigue, and increases with self-consciousness. The treatment of tic depends in a large measure on the proper recognition of the mental condition of the patient and the removal of the irritating cause.

To this category belongs another common affection ; STAMMERING AND STUTTERING.

Stammering is a bad habit, occurring in self-conscious, shy and other nervous persons, and once established it increases the original nervousness, so that the patient becomes still more afraid to speak. This constant fear and dread of speech failure is at the bottom of nearly all permanent stammering. Stammering and all speech defects are much worse when the patient is labouring under excitement. In ordinary conversation with friends the stammerer may have little difficulty ; but as soon as he begins to talk with those with whom he is unfamiliar, his speech defect becomes noticeable. When the others present are entire strangers and, above all, strangers whom he wishes to impress favourably, his stammering becomes pronounced. The mental element is the most important factor. Just as soon as consciousness of the task supervenes his power of co-ordination fails and stammering begins.

There are many systems to train people to overcome this speech defect. All of these systems have their successes and their failures. When the patient has confidence in the teacher and his method there is practically always quite a remarkable improvement at the beginning. Not infrequently after a month or so there is a tendency for the patient to drop back into old habits, discouraged as a consequence of loss of confidence. I have with very few exceptions succeeded in curing the defect by psychotherapy. The patient is put at ease and made to breathe properly, and, while in the relaxed state of ease and comfort, is made to forget any fears he may have and taught how to become less self-conscious and how to exercise self-control. The attention must be centred on something besides speech itself ; it must be so directed that he is unconscious of the co-ordination necessary for speech and so accomplishes it without difficulty. Even very bad cases have recovered under such treatment, which, of course, requires both patience and sympathy.

Mention should be made here also of the so-called OCCUPATION NEUROSES. These affections present one feature which is common to them all, namely, that certain actions, previously accomplished with perfect ease, are rendered difficult or even impossible in consequence of cramp, tremor, paralysis, or acute neuralgic pain, whereas other movements are performed by the same muscles without difficulty or discomfort.

As a matter of course, the upper extremities, and particularly the hands and fingers, are most liable to be thus affected, because these parts have more work thrown on them. The cases in which the lower extremities are involved are comparatively few in number. The most common examples are *writers' cramp* and *pianoforte players' cramp*.

WRITERS' CRAMP occurs almost exclusively as a sequence to worry, domestic or financial, in persons whose avocations require them to write for many hours daily. The majority of the sufferers are those who are compelled to write a good legible hand and overtax their muscles. Weakly subjects with a predisposition to nervous affections are most liable to be attacked, and when the symptoms have appeared they are apt to be aggravated by excesses of all kinds, and in fact, by anything which tends to lower the tone of the nervous system. In a considerable number of patients a cure has been effected by the use of galvanism, the application of which, however, must be adapted to each particular case.

Sometimes it is not a true inability but only a dread of inability to write. For example, I saw a clerk who wrote without difficulty when at home, but was immediately seized with cramp when he was obliged to write in his office. It was the presence of his superiors who sat in the same room which caused the attack. He recognised himself that in the presence of his chiefs the fear of not being able to write was the only cause of his helplessness.

Finally, though it is not strictly a functional disorder, I should like to say a few words on that terrible affliction—EPILEPSY. We distinguish principally two forms, one minor one—petit mal —in which the patient simply loses consciousness, and a major and more serious one—grand mal—in which the loss of consciousness is accompanied by convulsions and other symptoms. Those who have studied the subject most in recent years agree that the great majority of cases of epilepsy are not primarily due to acquired causes, but to some congenital defect, so that there is an inherent instability of the nervous system. This makes the patient liable to explosions of nerve force, figuratively speaking, boilings over of nervous energy, when not properly inhibited. Once such a paroxysm occurs it is likely to happen again, and very often it brings on gradual degeneration of the nervous system and of mentality. In many cases, however, this degeneration can be delayed or even completely prevented by putting the patient under favourable conditions. In recent years we have come to realise that epilepsy is more favourably influenced by a simple outdoor life in the country without worries and cares, with carefully regulated exercise in the open air, and special attention to the digestive tract, than by any formal remedial measures or drug treatment. The fewer the emotional storms, the less likelihood of repetitions of attacks of epilepsy. These patients need, above all, to realise that they cannot live the strenuous life nor even the ordinary busy life of most people. If they will but take this to heart and not attempt to engage in busy occupations, they may live quite happy lives ; and if mentally content and without worrying anxieties, they will have so few attacks as to incur only to a slight degree the dangers inevitably associated with fits of unconsciousness. When living a quiet placid life without worry about themselves or their concerns, the number of the epileptic attacks decreases in a noteworthy degree and the intervals between them become longer and longer. No medicine is so effective in prolonging the intervals between attacks as this placing of the patient in favourable conditions of mind and body. Our experience with the colony system has emphasised this fact. Considerable success has been

K

attained in suitable cases by "suggestion" treatment.

There is also a purely functional epilepsy—HYSTERO-EPILEPSY—consisting of convulsive fits in hysterical subjects, but this malady is rare in men.

CHAPTER IX

MENTAL INSTABILITY

THE SEMI-INSANE

IT may appear from a perusal of the previous chapters as if all men with an unstable nervous system were necessarily miserable. But this is by no means the case. There are people with an inherited nervous defect who are subject to periodical attacks of instability, in which, however, they are not only highly contented, but declare they feel better than ever and can accomplish more than they have ever been able to do.

Even perfectly healthy people of sound stock have their moods, being at one time happy and cheerful and better fitted for work, without any special cause, and at other times unhappy and depressed without being able to account for the change in their mood. One day we find an acquaintance emotionally elevated, gay, and full of projects, the next time we meet him he has the "blues," and in place of being lively he is taciturn and depressed. Ask him the cause of his exaltation, he can give no reason except that he feels unusually well. Many of us are also duller in the morning than in the evening; the early hours are filled with gloomy forebodings, which, as the day grows older, vanish and are replaced by a sense of well-being. Some people spend their lives in a seesaw between depression and pleasurable exaltation, contentment and discontentment. In some there is a periodic depression, in some periodic excitement, while in others the two mental states follow each other alternately. In the life of nearly every man or woman there are two periods of depression or exaltation which recur with a certain degree of regularity. These conditions often depend upon the state of physical health, the change of seasons, the amount of physical or mental work accomplished or to be done, or any one of a thousand intrinsic or extrinsic factors.

With reference to DEPRESSION, even a perfectly normal person under the influence of some sorrow may feel the memory of it renewed at every turn. It meets him when he awakens, and is with him when he goes to sleep. He cannot escape from its importunity, it crosses and obstructs his path, and often succeeds in diverting the logical current of his thoughts and actions. Such a state of mind is not, however, produced in a healthy subject, except in definite relation to some misfortune, nor does it continue indefinitely. But there are people who are born pessimists, who see everything from the dark side and derive no comfort from the mere pleasure of living. Sometimes they manifest a morbid suspicion of everything and everybody, and detect an interested or malicious motive in the most innocent actions of others, always looking out for an evil interpretation. Slight causes, external and internal, produce extraordinary depression with marked symptoms. The voluntary power is impaired, the patient is deprived of resolution, his will becomes paralysed and he is inactive ; he thinks slowly, he moves slowly, and this retardation applies to all his actions. There is a disinclination for work, even amusements are felt as nuisances. The subject finds no pleasure in anything, he shuns society, is averse to speaking, and when he does talk it is in regard to his personal condition. He is hypersensitive, broods over his real or fancied trouble, he suffers acute misery, and wishes he were dead.

Such is the depressed person, but there are others just as unbalanced, if not more so, whose

disorder results in an EXALTATION of all the
mental functions, creating a feeling of extraordinary happiness and well-being. Their good
spirits, except for an occasional slight abate-
ment, seem inexhaustible ; they make dangers
invisible, misfortunes light, life easy and its
struggle pleasant, with nothing but certain
triumph at its end. All the intellectual functions
are accelerated. There is a rapid flow of ideas,
so rapid sometimes that the patient cannot
express them quickly enough, and he may lose
the thread of conversation, or " run off the line,"
so to say, by introducing a great multitude of
non-essential accessory ideas, which both obscure
and delay the train of thought. His ideas may
get confused, or he may run to death one idea,
or have strange ideas which irresistibly force
themselves into consciousness.

Sometimes such patients have a wonderful
facility of expression and an inexhaustible
command of language. Not only so, but the
choice of phrases and words, the flow of conversation adorned by jests, anecdotes, and
pleasantries, varied according to their audience,
shows a mental brilliancy which is more often
than not quite unexpected and unlooked for in
the individual. They may be so brilliant
and witty that their friends remark what

good company they are, often without a suspicion that the increased vivacity is the result
of a morbidly excited nervous system. This
exuberance of thought, speech, and action,
which resembles that of the first degree of
drunkenness, ends by overcrowding and narrow-
ing the field of useful activity or of logical
thought. They sometimes possess the faculties
of imagination, invention, and expression in a
very high degree ; but the things they are lacking
in more or less completely are judgment, continuity and unity of direction in their intellectual
achievements and in all acts of life. The result
is that, in spite of certain superior qualities, these
individuals are incapable of behaving themselves
in a reasonable way and of regularly practising
any profession, even though it be below what
they would seem to be capable of. This is so
marked that it seems as though their whole life
had been nothing but a contradiction between
an apparent richness of means and poverty of
results.

Frequently these patients are not only extremely verbose, but will unburden their mind
even to chance acquaintances and undesirable
persons, and similarly they may write not only
incessantly but even to complete strangers.
At the same time it may be noticed that they

have lost the sense of proportion and of the fitness of what ought to be said or written. They are often petulant, they make no efforts to avoid being insolent, they join in discussions for which they are incompetent, pry into other people's affairs, fly into a temper for no just cause, and affect great sensitiveness on the subject of their honour. They take offence easily, are inclined to noisy arguing, and may even become violent without adequate cause. If they have followed hitherto a quiet mode of life, they may now seek frivolous society and the pleasures of the drinking saloon, and, in fact, give way to excesses which are beyond the limits of propriety and decency. The thing that characterises these subjects is a notable weakness, or even an entire lack of the power of control, of the superior brain over the passions and instinctive desires. The result is that they are the slaves of their passions and propensities.

These patients fear nothing. They feel better than ever, they do not want to consult a doctor or take the most elementary precautions, they are indifferent to their physical surroundings or hold them in contempt. They will take any risk and boast of it. They are optimists in every respect, and from optimism it is only a short step to ideas of pride and grandeur. Their

feeling of self-satisfaction and self-importance
is often so much increased that they will admit
only their own point of view and their own plans,
and in consequence of an overstimulated imagination they may think themselves underrated
geniuses. Indeed, for the time being, they may
have all the qualifications of the genius, except
the one of being able to materialise their ideas.
They lack the ability to do, as well as to contemplate. They may dream of revolutionising
the race with their ideas, but it never comes to
anything. In the pursuit of their extravagant
plans they completely lose sight of the realities
of life, keeping their gaze fixed only upon the
results, while they never take into serious consideration the difficulties and insufficiencies of
their methods. Yet, frequently, they hold to
their ideas, however unusual and absurd, till
everything is coloured and distorted by them.
Sometimes, however, the projects are as quickly
abandoned as they are formed, and embrace
spheres of labour and enterprise that are unknown and foreign to their experience. Others
are inclined to reckless speculations, or they buy
things they do not want, and therefore, if they
have the control over business affairs, financial
losses or other catastrophes are likely to be the
result.

The excitement of these patients is complicated by insomnia, but the sleeplessness is not exhausting or felt as unpleasant, and they suffer but little; on the contrary, they may exaggerate their power of resistance to sleep and boast of it. In order to occupy the long hours of wakefulness they concoct schemes and plan amusements and enterprises, into which they try to draw their friends and acquaintances. They allow themselves no time for resting, they have no time for proper meals at regular intervals, being driven about by constantly changing impulses or projects. In this condition they are sometimes very eccentric. They either have some peculiar habit, or wear some odd style of clothes, or have a queer manner of wearing their hair, or of walking, or writing, or speaking. The eccentricity is often shown by an imperious or obsessional tendency which drives the subject along some intellectual or moral line of action to the total exclusion of any useful or practical occupation.

After a few days or weeks the patient may return to his normal life, and if the attack was a mild one will feel none the worse for it, or if more serious he may brood over the follies he committed during the period of excitement. Some recover perfectly, in others the normal periods gradually shorten and chronic mental disorder may be the end.

Between attacks much can be done to ward off succeeding ones by so regulating the patient's life, occupation, and environment that excitement and strain are reduced to a minimum. Everything contributing to bodily and mental stress should be avoided as far as possible. Outdoor life in the country is the one most to be desired. Especially is it important that plenty of sleep is regularly secured. Hurry, worry, ambitious undertakings, indulgence in stimulants, things that reduce the bodily tone and harmony—all these are fruitful sources of recurrence. Wise supervision of the patient should be maintained by some competent person without the patient realising that it is being done. In severer cases treatment in a Mental Hospital, private or public, may be necessary.

CHAPTER X

THE EFFECTS OF ALCOHOL

THE DRINK AND DRUG HABITS

IN quite small quantities alcohol acts first of all as a stimulant, puts the person in an agreeable frame of mind, and fires the imagination, and gives vivacity to the conversation. That is why it is given at dinner-parties. It puts the guests in good humour, in a happy frame of mind, and makes them more attractive to one another. The stimulant effect does not last, however, it is only immediate. Alcohol soon ceases to have a stimulating effect and acts as a sedative, giving repose to the body and a quietness to the mind and conscience. It is to produce these latter results that it is taken by people in misery or trouble ; not as a stimulant, for then it would increase their sadness, but as a sedative to their feelings. Those persons who have not had a happy life find a glass of wine a pleasant companion ; it causes diminution of sensibility, drowns their trouble and grief, and if it does not give complete felicity and forgetfulness it dulls thought and obscures the painful feeling. They know that they may feel a little stupid, but they also know that all things they may view will appear in a rosier light. The man drinks because it makes him cheerful, modifies the course and colour of his ideas, and gives him forgetfulness or sleep. He has some disquietude or a troubled conscience, and the glass of wine or spirits puts him into an agreeable frame of mind, and modifies the course and colour of his ideas, and may even give him imagination, eloquence, and courage. Indulgence gives relief, but the danger is that the experiment may be repeated until it is not the pleasing sensation of intoxication that is craved after so much as an escape from sobriety which has become intolerable.

A list of reasons for imbibing was once given in *Punch*, which showed the absence of a guiding rule. One man took a glass because he was merry, and another because he was sad ; one man because a friend had come to see him, and another because his friend had left him ; one because he had a daughter married, and another because he had a daughter buried ; one because he had a rising, and another because he had a sinking ; and so on.

It is not of these minor and temporary causes

of which we wish to speak here, but of the deeper reasons for drinking which produce harmful effects and may lead the person to become a " drunkard " or " alcoholic." Not everyone who drinks, even to excess, is an alcoholic ; only those persons can be regarded as such who either continually or at certain periods suffer from a craving for alcohol.

All the reasons advanced by our temperance advocates have a good deal of truth in them, but would not drive a man to drink unless he were already a " weak character." He takes to drink, not so much from outward as from inward causes, by reason of his defective mental constitution. It is not everybody who can become a drunkard ; there must be a nervous predisposition, frequently hereditary. At the present day, when drunkenness is looked upon as disgraceful by the more educated classes, excessive drinking has vastly diminished. Total abstinence societies have been established for something like a hundred years, with the result that moderate people have become more moderate, and many moderate persons have become teetotalers. It is also probable that some mentally unstable persons have been saved by abstinence from becoming drunkards. But the actual number of habitual drunkards has not materially decreased in spite of all this temperance energy. It is fair, therefore, to conclude that, while unbalanced temperaments and instincts of self-indulgence are inherited, the actual way in which these instincts will manifest themselves depends upon the surrounding conditions which may happen to prevail.

Some people seem to think that craving for drink is created by the sight or presence of a public-house. Yet they have only to ask themselves how it is that they pass the public-house not only with indifference, but with loathing; and it will be borne in upon them that their contention is somewhat faulty. The truth is that nobody becomes a drunkard from choice or accident. Before a man takes to drink as a vice he has a taste for it, a predisposition which grows out of some physical defect, constitutional in the first instance, but liable to be aggravated by poor food, unwholesome surroundings, bodily wear and tear, and loss of moral tone.

Doubtless a few cases of alcoholism can be attributed solely to force of example, but even in these we must consider the brain disposition of the person upon whom the example exerts its influence. Several people may be thrown open to the same examples and temptations, and yet it is probably only the minority that succumbs, and is not this because of the different susceptibility or instability of the brains in question ?

Most liquors are taken for the sake of the effect and not because they taste nice. Indeed, to many people they are so nauseous that it requires a good deal of resolution to swallow them. To the temperate man and the abstainer drink offers no allurements, it satisfies no craving, it yields them no delight, and has for them no temptation. They are sober not because of their superiority of resistance, but they do not fall because, having no desire, they cannot be tempted. Many persons could not get drunk if they tried. They are drink proof, not because of any superior virtue, not because of any superiority of self-control, but because drink has for them no temptation. Others have such unpleasant sensations if they exceed a small quantity of alcohol that they are compelled to leave off long before they have taken enough to make them drunk.

It used to be thought that there was some subtle influence in beer or spirits which led those who begin by taking one glass to advance to two, ten, or twenty glasses. But closer observation has shown that it is only in the weak-minded that the habit of drinking creates a morbid desire for more drink, overcomes the will, blunts the moral sensibilities, and makes everything subservient to its demands, until the habitual intoxicating cup thrusts itself perpetually upon his thoughts, gradually occupying them so as to exclude all other ideas. The resistance and prayers of his friends are of no avail ; he declares he is driven by irresistible necessity to strong drink—" he will go mad without it."

I would recommend as an ideal standard that no one should drink or smoke before he is twenty-five years of age. After that total abstinence would be easy and certainly set a fine example. If there is the slightest tendency to excess it is the only way of salvation. If a man decides against total abstinence let him drink wine or light beer only, and drink no or only extremely diluted spirits. He should drink only once a day and that at dinner, or if he drinks more often, still only with meals. He should swear off solitary drinking, drinking between meals, drinking to seal a bargain, or to welcome a friend, or to pay for a service, or to join in or return a " round " of drinks when in company.

To no class of persons is intemperance more dangerous than to those inheriting an unstable nervous system. The researches of numerous investigators have shown that, speaking gener-

L

ally, the insane, the weak-minded, the epileptic, and those who have sustained grave head injuries are susceptible in unwonted degree to the evil influence of alcohol. Persons so afflicted are poorly equipped with power of resistance, either because of defective hereditary endowment, or because factors in their early development have rendered them unduly susceptible to toxic substances, so that they are profoundly affected by an amount that would only cause a mild exhilaration in a more stable organisation. For such unstable persons there can be no halfway course ; they cannot be temperate. *Such persons must be total abstainers.*

When alcohol is imbibed freely we have first of all slight excitement and a feeling of well-being, in which speech and gestures become more animated. There is at first a paralysis of the inhibitory apparatus, the loquacious stage, when the person becomes talkative, gay, and lively ; he thinks he is very funny and even witty, when perhaps he is uttering the most commonplace remarks, or reiterating the most fatuous statements. The general expression becomes one of silly self-satisfaction, with a fatuous smile, which may be blended with a look of astonishment. The ideas become crowded together and confused. The curb which fear of public opinion puts on the free expression of emotions and ideas, and the veil which hides the real moral disposition, are removed, whence the justification for the saying *in vino veritas*. There is interference with the processes of thought, ideas succeed each other so rapidly that there is no time to arrange them in orderly sequence. The emotions get unstable, the mood becomes, without any very obvious reason for the difference, gay, or sad, or full of tenderness. Whether the excitability will tend towards joy, melancholy, or anger depends on the environment ; the person laughs sometimes at the least little thing ; weeps, or grows sentimental or maudlin ; gets angry at the slightest cause. He may be argumentative and even pugnacious ; he may be profane, obscene, abusive, threatening, and may be violent. The exaggerated feeling of strength and well-being soon passes ; his movements are poorly controlled ; his gait becomes staggering and his speech thick.

So long as the person is seated he may speak and discuss subjects quite distinctly and rationally, and yet when he attempts to walk he may not be able to take one step, in fact, may not be able to stand. On the other hand, he may be able to walk quite steadily, yet be unable to articulate one word.

This particular stage of drunkenness often leads to considerable difficulty in police-court cases. For the person in this condition has lost control of the muscles of locomotion, but has control of the muscles in connexion with speech, and, having steadied himself against the counter, he can speak coherently and quite distinctly. The policeman having seen the staggering gait swears that the man was drunk; the bar-attendant, having heard the clear speech, declares the man was sober, otherwise he would not have supplied him.

A little later the conduct becomes more and more reckless; his smile a besotted grin; his intellect more and more dulled; a temporary paralysis may supervene, the person becoming insensible and unconscious. After sleep he wakens with headache, weakness, nausea, and loss of appetite.

It is related in an old rabbinical legend that after Noah had planted the vine that God had given him, Satan secretly watered it with the blood of a lamb, of a lion, and of a pig. The order in which these animals are named, though very likely without intentional significance, is interesting, for it corresponds roughly to the successive stages of acute vinous intoxication; first, the stage of mildly soporific euphoria;

secondly, that of noisy, garrulous, and actively quarrelsome excitement; and lastly, that of bestial and abandoned lethargy. It is during the second stage that a very large proportion of all crimes of violence are committed, and the sudden and often explosive appearance of this phase is not at first sight apparent.

ACUTE ALCOHOLISM generally follows excessive drinking in otherwise normal persons, but what may be excess to one person need not be so to the other. Persons suffering from shock, distress, physical disease, accidents, or any brain defect, temporary or permanent, and lastly, persons not accustomed to alcohol, may feel the effects of its intoxication after very small quantities, which would have no effect at all on the habitual drinker. Acute alcoholism generally develops suddenly. The chief mental characteristics of acute alcoholism are terror, mental distress, and confusion of ideas. Repugnant visual hallucinations are frequent and the patient may smell or taste poisons. Chief amongst the physical signs is a fine muscular tremor, most marked when the attention is distracted. If the movement is made rapidly the alcoholic may carry a glass to the mouth without spilling the contents, but if the attempt is made slowly the feat will be difficult of accomplishment.

The continued excessive use of alcohol has its effects on the nervous and mental health in other ways than in producing acute alcoholism. CHRONIC ALCOHOLISM shows itself in gradual and progressive mental deterioration and in certain physical changes that show the deplorable effects of the poison on the central nervous system and on the bodily organs and functions.

We have the ordinary public-house drunkard, one who begins his carouse in early morning ; he is found there as soon as the doors are opened. His loquacity as the day goes on becomes more and more intense, and he claims a certain familiarity with everyone he meets. At the close of the day he may or may not be quite intoxicated ; if he is so it is generally of the noisy or hilarious type, and probably will make night hideous by his noises.

The habitué of the West End club. This class of individual is very cantankerous, irritable, and infirm of purpose. He will remain in the smoking-room all day imbibing at intervals ; he is talkative to the various members and liable to be quarrelsome if contradicted or crossed in any way. Many of such cases ultimately suffer from loss of power of their limbs. He is a source of uneasiness to many of his friends, and his judgment in any matter requiring tact or discretion

is most deficient, and his advice when given
would probably do much more harm than
good if followed out, as his mind is fast
degenerating.

I now come to a type so often met with, that
of the self-satisfied alcoholic. He is not completely under its influence, and is able to control,
to a certain extent, his actions. He has a
familiar smile on his countenance, and is anxious
to tell strangers his private affairs. He will
insist upon shaking hands repeatedly, and though
his conversation is variable his mind will revert
to some small grievance which he will have
exaggerated into one of gigantic proportions,
and to which he will keep alluding, apparently
forgetting that he had previously done so ; a
partial loss of memory is here characteristic.

The mental enfeeblement is slow but progressive. At first the person feels unable to
apply himself to the tasks he formerly did with
ease ; his mind wanders ; he has a growing
sense of fatigue ; later he shows impairment of
judgment, poverty of ideas, and gradual failure
of memory. While forgetfulness is characteristic
of all forms of chronic alcoholism, the loss of
memory may be so prominent as to constitute
a special form of the disease. The characteristic
sign of this type of the malady is the instan-

taneous forgetfulness of events that have only just transpired. Thus names, or the simplest sentences, repeated over and over again to the patient, are totally forgotten either instantly or after the lapse of a few moments, nor does there exist any possibility of their recall in the future.

There is marked enfeeblement of the will, so that there is not the power, and often not the desire, to rise out of the rut of habit. Some of them honestly desire to lead a sober life, but fail in the struggle. This enfeeblement of the will-power is not confined to the inability of the patient to resist his alcoholic craving, but extends to other matters as well; so that he loses his power of initiative and of asserting himself, and becomes incapable of performing any work, except according to routine, and so becomes the tool of other people, by whom he is influenced and easily diverted from his purpose.

The person gradually undergoes a change in character; he becomes untruthful, loses his finer sense of honour, he—little by little—grows lax about things concerning which he was formerly most particular. He becomes indifferent to his own interests and regardless of the feelings or prosperity of his relatives and family. He sees those depending upon him suffering want and shame, yet pursues his downward course, seemingly indifferent to their needs or their entreaties. Sometimes he falls so low that he will pawn the clothing his wife has earned in order that he may procure money to buy more drink. Another striking feature is an unreasonable irritability, which frequently leads to outbreaks of passion of a blindly impulsive character, of which his family or his associates are often the victims. Wife-beating, inhuman treatment of children, attacks upon associates on the slightest provocation, are of daily occurrence during the stage of inebriety.

Along with these symptoms muscular weakness is apparent ; a fine tremor may come to be a pretty constant symptom, but coarser muscular twitchings also occur, and there is a painful condition of the nerves of the limbs, namely, neuritis. Frequent headaches, dizziness, difficulties in speech and gait are common, and convulsive seizures of an epileptoid character may appear. In the pronounced forms of chronic alcoholism we find a more decided blunting of common sensations. Chronic alcoholism often leads to insanity. Continuous inebriety tends also to bring about dilatation of the heart and lessen the vigour of the muscular movements of the stomach, which are necessary for good digestion.   It may also cause inflammation of the mucous membrane of the stomach, giving rise to nausea and vomiting.

One of the problems of the day is how to treat the dipsomaniac.   There are many chronic drinkers who recognise their danger and sincerely wish to be cured, more especially those who suffer from dipsomania at irregular intervals. When they regain normal consciousness they experience a feeling of profound despair and make the most solemn promises, perhaps actually drinking nothing but water, but in a few weeks or months the whole affair begins again.   These are the cases in which treatment by " suggestion " is successful.   The result has in many cases been astonishing.   So much attention has been given to the details of institutional care, and to the contending claims of the many medicinal agents which are supposed to have remedial virtues, that there has been some tendency to lose sight of the fact that the condition to be dealt with is at bottom a disorder of the will, and that it can only be really cured by restoring the patient's power of self-control.   Psychical treatment is so essential that even the best conceived physiological remedies will fail to do all that they should if they are not seconded by influences that act on the patient's mentality.

This point, which, of course, has to be considered in the treatment of practically all diseases, is naturally of the greatest importance in connexion with disorders where there is a predominant mental element. But it is not merely as affecting the action of medicines that this mental factor has to be taken into account ; it has an even more potent influence on the efficacy of treatment by restraint. When the weaning from the alcohol habit has been effected, not by re-education and restoration of the will, but by compulsion, this compulsion is very apt to excite a latent hostility which remains as a subconscious fixed idea to revive at some moment of weakness under the guise of a return of craving. This is undoubtedly the reason why restraint fails to produce a lasting cure in many cases of alcohol addiction, and it shows the extreme importance of accurate psychological study in dealing with patients of this sort.

The old method of treatment was to hypnotise the patient and then make post-hypnotic suggestions by telling the subject that when awake he would not desire or relish the drink to which he is addicted, or that his arm would be paralysed when he tried to raise the glass to his lips. These are not good suggestions, and I am not surprised that such patients after a time relapse into their old state. My method has always been to make a suggestion in harmony with the natural feelings of the patient, to make it seem that it is his own strength of will and not the effect of suggestion that has cured him of his habit. Having acquainted myself beforehand with his dominant propensities and controlling thoughts, his beliefs, prejudices, and mental environment, and having first secured his confidence, I then talk to him sympathetically in regard to the failing which he wishes removed. The best instincts have to be discovered and engaged. There is some element of good in every item of humanity, which can be elicited and drawn out. This means that the treatment must be individual. Sometimes it is effective to tell the patient that, when next he is tempted to drink, he will realise the awful picture he makes of himself and the disgust with which his wife and children, and all those whom he respects and holds dear, will observe him ; and that this scene will be so vivid before his eyes that he will experience no difficulty in withstanding the temptation. In all cases one must provide the patient with some strong counter-motive to break the habit and annul the recurrent craving. It is necessary, too, to enquire into and remove the exciting causes, to attend to the general nutrition of the body, and to see that the mind is occupied appropriately.

Patients addicted to the drink or other pernicious habit are readily cured by this method, the only condition being their willing co-operation.

THE MORPHIA HABIT

Second only in importance to alcohol, among the chemical poisons that produce a chronic intoxication showing psychical features, stands opium with its derivatives.

To some extent the notorious intolerance of the present generation to pain is largely responsible for the increase, a toothache or a neuralgia being sufficient cause or excuse for the sufferer to fly to morphine, or some other narcotic, for relief. It is of the greatest importance to recognise that the anodyne and soothing properties of opium are peculiarly seductive to some individuals, and are apt to be sought long after the causes which led to its employment have passed away. What happens is this : the patient has become accustomed to his dose and awaits it so soon as the effects of the last one have passed off. He tells us of vague pains and miserable feelings which appear to demand recurring doses, but these feelings are commonly nothing more than the pains of craving for fresh intoxication, a habit having already set in. Hence the extreme unwisdom of permitting nurses or relatives to administer opiates or give hypodermic doses of morphine at their discretion in any case.

The victims of the drug habit are, as a rule, addicted to the practice of it in secret, and take infinite pains, with supreme subtlety, to hide it from their nearest and dearest relations. This fact indicates a measure of shame and a recognition of the fact that their habit is one which, if known, would entail reprobation, and possibly ostracism, in their social surroundings, together with the institution of measures to put a stop to the indulgence. The habit of morphinism is readily detected on stripping the patient by the scars of numerous punctures, especially on the left arm.

The first effect of morphia is to make one think quickly and clearly, but this soon passes away and a dreamy state supervenes. Persons who continue the use of morphia fail to get the acute effects, but they are held in its power because of its ability to exhilarate them temporarily, enough to make them forget their troubles. They find to their dismay, however, that in order to get this result they must increase the quantity of the drug and repeat the dose oftener. It is not that the patient has a pleasure in drug-taking, but that it is heaven for him to have the drug as it is hell to be without it. No physician should ever place a hypodermic syringe, or a prescription for morphia, renewable at will, in the hands of his patient with instructions how to use it.

The permanent effect upon the faculties in those instances in which the abuse of the drug has been long continued, or the amount taken excessive, is shown in impairment of memory and lessened ability to apply one's self to physical or mental work. The stability of the emotions is conspicuously affected. Persons indulging in morphia are easily dejected and irritated.

Anxiety, especially at night, is often experienced. These patients often complain of numbness, or hypersensitiveness; their pupils are usually contracted, their gaze is often furtive or staring; they are usually pale, with marked pallor of lips or ears. Some of them get hypochondriacal; some become weak and tremulous, lose flesh, suffer from dizziness, fainting spells, profuse perspiration and palpitation.

The moral nature undergoes grave changes, as shown in pronounced moral obliquities, and in the resort to any means, no matter how unscrupulous, even actual forgery and theft, to obtain the drug. The idea of personal responsibility falls to the lowest ebb ; thought, action, and even the most imperative duties are shunned. While the largest numbers of these unfortunates are not insane in the stricter sense of the word, there is always present a certain degree of ethical obliquity, irritability, peevishness, and moroseness. They lie unblushingly. It is never safe to believe the word of a morphio-maniac ; his conscience is obtunded and he will prevaricate with or without reason.

In order to cure the drug habit we must treat the patient rather than the habit. He must be braced up, must be made to understand that if he wants to quit the habit, no matter how slavishly he is addicted to it, he can do so. The first and absolutely necessary preliminary of the treatment is to lift up the patient in his own eyes and make him understand that, low as he has sunk, his case is not hopeless, that his degradation is not at all uncommon nor so rare as he might think, and that men and women have succeeded in lifting themselves out of conditions worse than his. If mild tonics are applied for a time so that the symptoms due to the physio-

logical effects of the excessive use of the drug
are minimised, treatment by " suggestion " can
then be used on the lines described under treatment of the drink habit.   Excellent results have
been thus achieved.

CHAPTER XI

THE "CHANGE OF LIFE" IN MAN

THAT the physiological changes in the female sexual organs during the "change of life" are often accompanied by definite nervous and mental disorders is universally known. But that the changes in the glandular structure of man during the same period also give rise to similar disorders, though not in the same degree, has hitherto attracted little attention. As a rule, no notice is taken of the "change of life" in man, but there are many men in whom at this period nervous and mental disturbances do occur similar to those in women, only that in the female sex they are severer and attention is drawn to them because of the cessation of the menses. Nearly every man between 45 and 55 years of age becomes conscious of a change in his feelings and character as well as in his bodily state.

The "change of life" affects profoundly, more in some, less in others, the entire constitu-

tion, mental and physical. Nature is kind to the
majority and imperceptibly prepares the system
for the change, so that they pass through it with
comparatively little trouble. With some the
change is so gradual as not to be taken particular
notice of, with others the change is more or less
abrupt. A man, hitherto full of energy, enthusiasm, and cheerfulness, discovers that the
pleasures of life no longer offer the same enjoyment to him, that the society of younger men is
apt to bore him, that they belong to a new
generation, whose interest and enjoyments are
no longer his own. His views, political, social,
or scientific, for which he has hitherto fought
with all his energy, become moderated. He sees
the defects of reform movements, if not their
utter hopelessness. His entire conduct is now
more influenced by reason than by emotional
impulse. He gets more domesticated. His
family has an increased interest for him. Altogether he has grown more serious and sedate,
but he and his friends think this is only natural
with the advance of years, and trouble no
further about it.

One of the chief constitutional symptoms is a
tired condition, often implying an instinctive
feeling that work, exertion, and effort are not
always entirely worth the doing. Physiologically

and psychologically, energising by itself is no longer felt to be so necessary. The tired feeling often leads to a lowering in the desires and ideals. Pleasures that cost little and imply small exertion are preferred to pleasures of the higher sort that need some strenuousness to attain them. Bad habits begin to show their cumulative effects, and the recovery after indiscretions is less certain and slower. There is a slackening of the intellectual powers with inability to concentrate the attention and diminished energy for work. The intellectual processes are both retarded and more difficult. There is no longer the same intuition and inspiration and former concentration. In intellectual workers the imaginative power is diminished, hence it is difficult for them to originate new work. In consequence they become dissatisfied with their occupation and lose self-confidence. It can be noticed that they get easily irritated, that they get easily dissatisfied and are addicted to grumbling, in short, that nothing pleases them. They are impatient of opposition. They are easily provoked to anger, even by persons they love. Family events, the theatre, music and the sight of misery excite their feelings to an unusual extent. In one word, their tendency is to become " effeminate." Many patients complain, in addition, of

what is commonly called " stage-fright." The
brilliant orator, the distinguished performer, the
proud speculator now dread public assemblies,
or when engaged in their respective avocations
come suddenly to a standstill. Their memory
fails them, they forget what they intended to
say, or play, or reckon. After one or more
experiences of this nature they are overcome by
chronic fear; dreading some misfortune, they do
not know of what kind, they can only say that
they feel they will always be helpless or ill.
The diminished capacity for work makes them
fear poverty. In consequence of their anxieties
sleep is disturbed, although genuine insomnia is
the exception. Sleep is uneasy, less deep, and
consequently less refreshing than formerly. The
subject has to coax somnolence and resorts to
various devices to gain his object. He becomes sad and depressed ; he feels the burden
of responsibility weighing heavily upon him,
perhaps that life has been somewhat of a failure
and that he has accomplished very little in spite
of all he has tried to do ; the " love of life " is
diminished, and not infrequently attempts are
made at self-destruction, which take the family
all the more by surprise since no real motive
can be found to account for such conduct. This
state is associated with a peculiar sensitiveness

to the action of alcohol and tobacco, which even in reduced quantities give rise to distressing sensations. More or less persistent headache is a common feature. Already noticeable on awakening in the morning, it is apt to get worse as the hours go by, and ere the day's work is over it may assume a throbbing character. It is specially apt to be caused or intensified by intellectual effort, by alcohol, or by excitement of any kind. The freshness of the complexion is lost, the skin has grown darker and rougher, the face begins to show wrinkles, the lustre of the eyes is fading, the various bodily organs get fatigued more quickly and require more rest than hitherto, and when worked to excess painful sensations are apt to follow. The sexual desire as well as potency is diminishing and sexual hypochondriasis is not uncommon.

At the same time, the defence against disease is lowered and often this is the beginning of the end, the time when the first signs of that illness sets in, to which in after years the man succumbs. For both sexes, the climacterium is a period for the readaptation of the bodily machinery to a more modified functional activity. If at this period there are cares and sorrows, mental or physical over-exertion, it will be more difficult than ever to retain the elasticity. At any other time the body would have recovered easily. Now there is not enough vitality and nervous energy, or only after a period of long inactivity.

In order to cure the physical and psychical disturbances accompanying the male climacterium, we must treat the nervous system. The success is striking. Most of the cases recover their former health and energy in a very short time. It is by strengthening the nerve centres that we accomplish a cure, not by local stimulation. Electricity does wonders in such cases. It has the effect of a general tonic in conditions of debility and exhaustion. It regenerates the nerve-force, increases the vitality, and gives resistance to disease. It is a thousand pities that its practice should be left so largely in the hands of quacks.

The patient must be made to realise that if his body has lost in elasticity it will now gain in massive strength, that if his thought-engine throbs with less violent pulsation it will now gain in cool, orderly and harmonious vibrations, and that sound maturity can be quite as efficient and enjoyable, though not so exuberant, as youth. It is no use sighing for days that have gone ; he must enjoy the glory and triumphs of manhood without regrets for the past or fears for the future.

He should keep up his exercises and recreations and not drop any of his outdoor interests unless he can acquire other ones in their places. So long as he likes to take active exercise and sport and feels exhilarated and refreshed by them, he should keep them up. When he feels that they are getting a little too much for him, when he does not feel fresher for them next day, he should cut them down a little in intensity.

Much the same principles apply in the matter of eating. He should follow his appetite, checked by the results of his personal experience. As the old saying runs, a man at forty is " either a fool or a physician " in the matter of diet. He has usually found out for himself what kinds and amount of food agree with him and what do not. Most men after forty-five, or certainly after fifty, will notice a slight but distinct falling off in appetite. This is a hint that the body cannot utilise as much food as before, and should be acted upon.

Obesity at this age is not a disease, but in nine cases out of ten a normal healthful process, a laying-by of capital against the evil days that are coming. Fat laid on after forty-five is usually lost before seventy, and is neither a sign nor a cause of disease, " Anti-Fat " advertisements to the contrary notwithstanding.

Unfortunately, shortly after the age at which this deposit of fat-surplus occurs the body engine is apt to show signs of wear and tear, and original defects in tubing, boiler, steam gauge, and gearing reveal themselves under the strain ; but it is not the first change that causes the second. The dreaded fatty degeneration of the heart and liver has nothing whatever to do with general increase in body weight, however generous. It occurs more often in the emaciated than in the obese. Therefore let no one hesitate to laugh and grow fat, or starve himself for fear the " fat will get round his heart." Nearly all weight-reducing diets and treatments reduce strength also and are dangerous if long persisted in. Fatness is perfectly compatible with the highest grade of efficiency.

Next as to sleep : the man at this period of life should take plenty. Time spent in sound sleep is never wasted. The man of middle age will find that he cannot take quite as much sleep as formerly ; he tends to wake earlier and more easily, but this should make him the more insistent to take all that he possibly can. He cannot stand the loss of sleep as he once did. If he has been up till the small hours he is more apt to feel ill-effects of it next day.

A great point is to keep up variety in mental

occupations and to keep up the interest in many things so as to prevent early mental torpor. Exclusive devotion to work has the result that amusements cease to please ; and when recreation becomes imperative, or is the only thing left as in old age, life becomes dreary from lack of its sole interest—the interest in business. The man of middle age must not plan too soon retirement from business unless he has a hobby or another pursuit to retire on, as well as a competency. If he is so unfortunate as to have no hobby, by all means let him beg, borrow, or hire one. Better still, two, one indoor and one outdoor. The hobby should be commenced while he is still at active work, since the inclination and aptitude to begin something new becomes increasingly difficult as one grows older. The exercise of the brain in intellectual pursuits keeps that organ, and with it the entire body, young, and business men would do well to choose some intellectual hobby. It is highly instructive to observe the longevity in men of high intelligence. They usually are or have been engaged in those callings which require the continued exercise of the intellectual faculties upon comparatively new matter, or upon new combinations of familiar data.

CHAPTER XII

GENERAL TREATMENT OF NERVOUS DISORDERS

HYGIENIC PHYSICAL MEASURES

MANY a patient suffering from a milder form of nervous disorder feels better for a " change." A short release from his burdening duties, a break in the monotony of his work, often does wonders. He should seek conditions and influences which give fair chances for the recuperation of his energies, and which are adapted to his abilities, his knowledge and social condition, and are full of joyful associations and emotions.

Patients suffering from a severer form of nervous disorder have frequently to be recommended to take absolute REST for a time, to withdraw completely from the occupation, whether it be of business or pleasure, which has exhausted their nervous system, and from the source of worry which has depressed their mentality. Speaking generally, such separation

171

is beneficial for the patient when those living with him display either exaggerated tenderness or disobliging indifference, or an irritating want of comprehension of his feelings of malaise and his sufferings. In such case he is better isolated from his family and those surroundings in which his ailment developed or which helped to make it chronic. In withdrawing from his habitual circles the patient further escapes the often too attentive care of his relatives and the incessant questions about his health, or one symptom or another of his complaint, with which they overwhelm him ; he breaks away, so to speak, from that moral atmosphere made up of solicitude and commiseration, and sometimes also of ironical indifference, by which his mental depression and the irritability of his temper have been fostered.

In the milder cases complete rest from work is not to be recommended ; they will do better by cutting down their obligations. Complete rest is likely to make them less able for work, to diminish their fitness instead of increasing it. For the one thing which requires an expenditure of energy is the setting in motion. This alone is painful. The wise simply manage so as to be always in motion. The man who does not work regularly and without interruption is constantly obliged to renew the setting in motion, to compel

his brain to become attentive, to constrain his
intellect by command to a given task, and this
the most gifted find fatiguing. Still there are
some brain workers for whom the perfection of
a holiday will be found in doing nothing, in the
simple contemplation of nature : the sight of
the sea, of the forest, of the country. This
razes from their minds the manifold associations
and stimuli of their ordinary lives.

So-called " rest-cures " are often beneficial to
those whose nervous systems are greatly exhausted, but there are few patients so seriously
ill that they require to stay in bed all day ; and
I have known a good many who were rendered
so irritable and restless by " rest in bed " that
their condition was worse after the " cure "
than at the commencement of the treatment.
It has to be remembered that, if we isolate the
patient, we place him under artificial conditions
and cannot judge of his real progress ; for he will
have to return to those surroundings which
brought about his neurosis.

Sometimes the patient tries TRAVELLING as a
remedial measure in the hope that it may do
him good. It is quite true that a change of
scene and surroundings, combined with relief
from work, is very beneficial in diverting the
patient's thoughts from himself and restoring

him to a healthier frame of mind. But again, a physician's advice is required; for we have to remember that a nervous patient is frequently not only jaded in mind and body, and unable to stand the strain of travelling or to take an interest in sight-seeing, but he is also suffering from digestive derangements and sleeplessness, and these latter conditions are often aggravated by travelling. He should not start off on a sea voyage before his physical condition has improved, for not for everyone is the life on board a ship suitable, certainly not in a case of mental depression. Life on board ship is in itself—by its monotony and want of interest—depressing to many travellers, and it is rarely that a ship's doctor has had any special experience of nervous disorders. We see sometimes evidences of the non-success of this mode of self-help in the newspaper paragraphs, which chronicle the accidents to persons when taking sea voyages for their health. There is no objection, however, to a patient going on a sea voyage when still fairly fit or during the period of convalescence.

A holiday is an event in the spiritual life, and in proportion as we have or have not the gifts of the spirit, so we enjoy a holiday, or fail to enjoy it. The very words we use of a holiday proclaim its spiritual significance; for we call it a change, or recreation—that is to say, conversion, or regeneration.

Peace of mind, readiness to please and be pleased, simplicity and reverence are factors of a holiday no less essential than fresh air, exercise, sight-seeing, and sport. But this peace of mind, though it thrives well on solitude and silence, thrives likewise on a great crowd in a strange city. It needs only to be free ; it must have the liberty of the spirit of holidays. One of us finds that freedom in the loneliness of the country, another finds it in the companionship of unfamiliar fellow-creatures ; there is no accounting for what we falsely call tastes, but are in reality diversities of gifts. One word of advice : the holiday-maker should not take with him the same clothes and talk which he has been using all the season.

There is a conviction in the minds of many people that in matters regarding the recuperation of health there is nothing like the SEA. " A blow from the briny " is a very common recommendation in cases of slackness, and is meant to suggest that sea air is salutary. In not a few cases this is a delusion. It is true that as a rule there is nothing to be said against the quality of sea air ; it is cool, pure, and clean, its supply is unlimited and ever fresh ; yet it is not always that the individual seeking strength can respond to the powerful and exciting stimulus of the bracing sea air; the digestive, secretory, circulatory, and eliminatory systems may be goaded to an energy of which they are incapable by reason of a general debilitated condition; they are not able to do their work without exhaustion, and the last state may be worse than the first. When sea air disagrees with the temperament digestive disturbances arise; and if the excretory functions are not in good going order, as in the case of the so-called bilious individuals and plethoric persons, headaches, giddiness, and a train of other symptoms make an appearance. As a rule the effect upon such cases of the less stimulating country air is magical. When that is so, it means that the great human machine and its complexes gain vigour best by repose. When strength has been restored in this way, the tonic air of the sea may then be tried with the greatest advantage. There can be no more satisfactory formula for the restoration of the hard-worked person than first a soothing, restful environment at home or in the country and then a tonic one of sea or mountain air. To plunge straight into the tonic, invigorating air of the seaside is an irrational procedure for many "run-down" cases.

Then as to BATHING, its chief value lies in its exhilaration. It does not do to make a penance of it. Not all persons can enjoy it, and to some it does positive harm. One may be clean without bathing. The benefit derived from the morning bath is in the reaction, the glow that follows it, not in the cold plunge itself. Cold in general, and cold water in particular, are superb tonics, first to the nervous system, through its branches in the skin, second to the heart and blood-vessels as shown in the glow, and third to the muscles and digestive glands. But, like any other tonic, while a small dose stimulates, a large one depresses; and the size of the dose depends entirely on the bather. For a strong, vigorous man or woman in the prime of life, nothing is better than the cold plunge. It is the reaction that we should aim at. If we do not get this the bath is a failure, if not an injury. For persons less vigorous, the temperature of the bath should be modified to a degree which enables one to lie in it for at least half a minute with comfort; for the shock of sudden cold has its dangers, especially after fifty, when the arteries are losing their elasticity. The best temperature is the one that gives the best reaction, and consequently most pleasure, and all baths should be taken in a reasonably warm room.

N

As in the cold bath, so there is no benefit gained by heroically enduring chilliness, shivering, and acute discomfort in sea water, under the impression that because it is disagreeable it is manly and bracing and will in the long run do good. Sea bathing should be regarded solely as an enjoyment, and practised as such. The strong will find it a bracing and exhilarating sport, and may indulge in it freely, not only without harm, but with great benefit. The weak and relaxed and under-vitalised, and especially all who know themselves to be below par in any respect, should indulge in it most sparingly.

As regards hot baths, these also have their uses and their drawbacks. They have two distinct purposes of utility, the purely mechanical one of cleansing, the other for just the opposite function of the cold bath, soothing and relaxing instead of toning up and invigorating. The relaxing and soothing effects of the hot bath are very real, and, under proper circumstances, of great value. Partly by virtue of its heat, partly by the steam which is inhaled in the course of it, and partly by its stimulating effect upon the excretory glands of the skin, the hot bath has a remarkable effect in removing aches and pains, or " taking the soreness out of " tired muscles.

For these purposes it should obviously be taken at or near bedtime, when the day's work is over, and the skin may safely remain relaxed for at least one to three hours afterwards. For the average man or woman a bath of this description taken in the evening is perfectly legitimate and, indeed, a beneficial procedure. It has also usually the desirable effect of inducing sleep in those who are disposed to insomnia.

However, it may become a source of danger by its very attractiveness. It is soothing and so enjoyable that it is easy to carry it to such an extreme as to relax the skin and produce a more or less permanently depressing effect on the nervous system by its overuse.

Then as regards MUSCULAR EXERCISE. Undoubtedly, a man who works hard with his mind feels better for a few moments of physical exercise ; remaining fixed in one's chair at a desk is not a healthful practice. But physical exercise is advantageous only if it be moderate ; otherwise it simply adds to the fatigue of the brain. Prolonged and fatiguing exercises, taken not for any enjoyment in them, but, as a matter of conscience, "to build muscle," are distinctly dangerous. The heaviest strain of exercise is thrown not on the muscles, but on the heart and blood-vessels. Training should be directed to the

nervous system. The mere increase in strength
of a particular muscle counts for little. It is the
rapid, accurate, purposeful combination of a
dozen muscles with the eye, the ear, the sense
of touch and resistance that forms two-thirds of
training. And this is done solely through the
nervous system.

One must not look at exercise merely for its
effect on the muscular apparatus. Its psychological value is as important as its physiological.
People often take up home gymnastics with
religious enthusiasm and get splendid results
out of them—for a time. Few keep it up long.
That does not mean that the exercise system is
at fault. It simply means that it failed to
hold the interest. If a man forces himself to
exercise simply because he thinks it his duty,
more than half its benefits are lost. For a really
valuable exercise is one which reaches beyond
the muscles and the digestive organs ; it braces
up and stimulates the mind. The kind of exercise that hits the mark is the kind a man likes
for its own sake.

There are many people who keep well and who
do their work successfully without ever taking
any formal exercise at all. A man who takes an
intelligent interest in the character of his food, who
eats properly, attends to the demands of his

bowels, keeps his skin in good order, and provides himself with a decent amount of mental relaxation—such a man can often go for a long time without any special exercise.

But a man who eats big dinners must have bodily exercise. So must a man who works in a badly ventilated room. So must a man who has a tendency to worry, or to constipation, or to headache. Indeed the number of those who escape the need is very small.

It is the quality of muscular effort that counts rather than quantity. So long as muscular effort is strengthening the heart and developing the nervous system and increasing the appetite, it is doing good ; beyond this it is physiologically valueless, often harmful, however great an economic or sporting value it may have. So long as exercise gives pleasure, exhilaration, it is doing good. When it is not enjoyed, it is either neutral or harmful physically. Some men cannot do without a considerable amount ; others keep " fit " with little or none.

For men of middle age exercise is necessary but difficult to prescribe, for they have not the speed for quick games, nor the suppleness for gymnastics ; yet they eat and drink more, and more richly, than the young, for the pleasures of the table outlast others, and, seeking neither fame among men nor love of women, they sit long over meat and wine.

Old age needs little exercise ; sunshine and good company cheer the old man. He needs restraint more than incentive. We must see that the old man's machinery works with as little friction as possible.

A word of warning as to intermittent excesses in the way of exercise may not be out of place. Men who lead a sedentary life rush off to the country for the week-end and play golf or tennis, or take long walks all the time, returning to town on Monday feeling the reverse of " fit." They have, in fact, fatigued their muscles with work to which habitual inaction has made them unequal, and the result is that they are poisoned by an excess of waste products, engendered by the unwonted exertion. Exercise needs to be conducted with care ; it is not at all times good, nor in all degrees. Many suffer from lack of it, but many from taking it indiscreetly.

Walking is perhaps the best and most readily available form of exercise for most people, but has one disadvantage. As soon as the walk becomes too much of a routine, and the ground gone over has lost its interest, or is even of such a nature as to permit introspection or occupation with other things, rather than with the surroundings, then walking loses most of its efficacy as a form of exercise. That is probably why people find golf such a healthy exercise. They get a walk while at the same time their thoughts are centred on the game with its endless varieties, and they can be so absorbed in it that for the time they cannot think of anything else ; and for the class of patient we are speaking of this is just what is necessary for them.

Exercise should be allied with pleasure ; it is for recreation. The mere motion to a place is not enough, unless to move is gladness simply ; as oftentimes it is in sunshine for the beauty of it and in storm for the pleasure which the contest gives. A man will say he takes enough exercise, because rising late and eating a full meal in too short a time he walks at top speed to his station or his office ; another, because when exhausted with the day's work he forces himself to walk a long way home. The one hurries, the other fatigues himself ; neither effort is the exercise that brings health, but a strain that often causes disease. So it comes that there is a philosophy of exercise, and its practice should be varied to each age and condition of life.

The patients whom we have under consideration often fail to appreciate the nervous and mental origin of their numerous complaints and

seek MEDICINAL AID for their individual symptoms, whether it be headache, backache, pains
in the limbs, dyspepsia, palpitation, insomnia,
and the rest. They seem to suppose that the
drugs fit diseases in a perfect way. The physician
does not always give drugs because he thinks it
will cure the disease; he has to give a prescription sometimes because the patient is not
happy till he gets it; too often he is not happy
even then. The popular belief in the all-sufficing
efficacy of drugs is widespread. The aristocratic
patient no more believes that his disorder can
be cured without the aid of a prescription than
his poorer fellow-mortal, who, when ill, attends
regularly at the hospital or dispensary in order
to obtain the bottle of physic, which he looks
upon as indispensable to the restoration of his
health. The popularity of the bottle depends
upon the basal idea that in some mysterious way
it represents the doctor's intelligence and skill
in a form capable of being swallowed, and so
brought into direct contact with the disease.
There are numberless occasions when drugs are
given, there being at the time no distinct indication for giving any, but the sick are not reasonable
beings, and, unless they have a bottle of medicine
to anchor their faith to, they are in a state of
unrest that is positively harmful to their pro-

gress. But there are multitudes who are not in this parlous state, who are capable of listening to reason; but having been taught to look for their prescription or their bottle of medicine, they have no idea of the value of advice only or of the need of the watchful eye. It is very disappointing when, after we have been giving advice for about an hour and flattered ourselves on having made an impression, we are met with the question on leaving : " Are you not going to give me a prescription ? "

The advance of civilisation has done little or nothing to decrease the hopeful spirit which throughout the ages has prompted man to believe in the curative power of drugs. No doubt, the cut-and-dry method of prescribing in the outpatient departments of hospitals is responsible to some extent for the implicit belief in the physic bottle. The patient wishes for cure and immediate relief ; he or she believes that the physician who has studied so much has some remedy already prepared for such disease, and all that he will have to do is to go to the pharmacist and get it. He listens only distractedly to the counsels on hygiene which the serious physician gives him, and he looks upon them merely as measures intended to favour the medicinal action, which no doubt they often are.

The general idea of treatment amongst the public seems to be that certain preparations relieve certain symptoms, and that when particular phenomena present themselves the same remedies must be used, no matter what the origin of these symptoms. Slight ailments, vague aches and pains, are borne with a varying amount of patience by different individuals. In many, the least departure from health is a signal for the self-administration of drugs. Taking drugs without consultation with a medical practitioner is undoubtedly on the increase, and it is the delight of some individuals to advise their friends to take certain things for the relief of their ills. Many of the popular preparations are of course harmless, only containing simple ingredients; but when more potent remedies are used, such as narcotics, the risk becomes serious.

It is very common for patients when they suffer from nervous exhaustion or are " run down " to ask a physician for a " tonic," and often they get it. This is a mistake, for many of the nervous symptoms due to exhaustion require a " sedative " medicine and not a tonic. Tonic remedies may be given when the tremors, palpitation, morbid fears, etc., have disappeared; then they will prevent a relapse, but to give

them in the early stage frequently aggravates
the patient's condition.

Certainly, we must raise the vital energy of
the patient, but the physician must choose the
proper time for it. There is a great difference
in vital energy. One man has more of it than
another. One man recovers rapidly and surely
after a nervous breakdown, while another drags
along through years of semi-invalidism. Functional nervous disorder is due to an enfeeblement
of nerve force, and to this the treatment must
be directed as well as to the mental symptoms.
A valuable agent for raising the tone of the
nervous system, the resisting power, and the
general vitality of the patient is ELECTRICITY.
There are several reasons why electricity
has been tardily established as a therapeutic
agent. Until recently there was a great lack
of precision in the knowledge possessed concerning it. Besides this, electricity has always
appealed to the human imagination, and in the
hands of quacks and charlatans has been utilised
to impress that large section of the public which
is gullible ; but with the effect of raising the
distrust and prejudice of medical men against
a therapeutic measure for which marvellous
powers were claimed. Lay practitioners may
understand the machine which they are using,

and have some general knowledge of electricity; but they know little or nothing of the anatomy and physiology and the diseases of the nervous system. Because electrical treatment fails to do any good in these cases, and sometimes does positive harm, there is a prejudice against the treatment not only on the part of the public, but also on the part of a good many medical men who have not studied nervous diseases very closely, and have never been called upon to give electrical treatment. On the other hand, physicians who do know all about the good effects of electricity have been too much in the habit of recommending lay practitioners, over whom they can have little or no control. Even if the electricity is applied in accordance with the instructions received, there is the mental element in all nervous disorders which must never be neglected, and none but a medical man can be a skilled psychotherapist. The consequences of electrical applications in the hands of non-medical persons may be disastrous. When we think of it, a man or woman who has taken a three months' course in some hospital or quack medical institution can set up in practice for himself, and advertise electrical treatment in competition with men who spent five or six years in their medical education and several years more in getting skilled in their specialty.

Gradually the utilisation of electricity is passing out of the hands of pretenders and showmen, and its value and merit are becoming recognised by thoughtful men and scientific workers, who see in it a vast power for good if kept within the compass of its applicability. Medical electricity has been undergoing very important developments during the last few years, and to an extent scarcely realised by those who are not intimately associated with the subject. It is now much more scientifically understood, and electrical applications are correspondingly more accurate and reliable. The day has gone past when a more or less intelligent manipulation of a few switches was considered a sufficient qualification for the practice of electro-therapeutics. The best results will be obtained only by those whose medical and scientific training has been comprehensive.

Often the nervous system is too exhausted for the patient to respond to psychotherapeutic influence. When by electrical, medicinal, or other treatment we have improved his general constitutional condition, he feels " fit " again, and his morbid fears or other abnormal feelings disappear without any special effort. On the other hand, where they are more deeply rooted, the patient's attendances for electrical treatment give us an opportunity—which we might not get otherwise—of employing such "suggestion" therapy, persuasive and analytical methods, as may suit his individuality, and thus both his mental and physical health are restored.

CHAPTER XIII

THE POWER OF SUGGESTION IN DAILY LIFE
AND MEDICAL PRACTICE,
AND OTHER METHODS OF PSYCHOTHERAPY

It is a popular error that SUGGESTION is practised only by medical men, and chiefly as hypnotic suggestion. We cannot escape its influence. First of all, there are the subconscious elements of our character which act on us as a constant suggestion, fashioning, after their own image, all our impressions and all our thoughts. Every man, of necessity, sees other men and Nature itself through the prism of his own individuality. Thus the wicked man believes in the wickedness of others, and the pessimist is convinced deeply that everything is wrong, when only himself is wrong. On the other hand, there are people who scarcely ever act from motives originating within themselves, but whose entire lives are lived in obedience to the suggested ideas and feelings of others. The feelings of affection, esteem, awe, or fear, which those who are talking to us inspire in us, surreptitiously prepare the paths of our understanding, and our reason is often taken in a trap. Somebody's optimistic reflection can give us strength, and, on the other hand, his ill-humour can take away all our enthusiasm and energy. Some individuals seem to have a " winning way " with them, and are able to induce others to fall into their way of thinking and to do for them what they wish done. We let ourselves be captivated by their superficial eloquence, by the charm of their language. Even the most resolute characters are influenced by suggestion. It is only required that the suggestion should be made artfully. The idea need only be introduced discreetly and gradually in order to succeed. By indirect suggestion, the subject has no consciousness that his views are being modified. Besides, an idea introduced almost unnoticed is likely to lie latent for a period, and, when it does assert itself, it will appear to the subject to have been originated by himself.

Children are trained almost wholly by suggestion. Next to the parental influence, the suggestions received during school life have the greatest influence on the formation of the future character. Suggestion lies at the bottom of all forms of moral and religious teaching. It is, in fact, the basis of education. We are all open to suggestion, but some are more so than others. The maintenance of social life depends to a great extent on the degree of power of making and receiving suggestions; and the firmest friends and the happiest couples in life are frequently those who are in this respect well matched. The measure of pleasure we get from life depends more on our suggestibility than on any other factor. Some people can be happy even in misery. Books are often bought because of their suggestive titles; fashionable clothes are worn because of the suggestion of wealth and respectability. Certain foods, the habit of open or closed windows, and other idiosyncrasies and whimsies often produce the pleasures of comfort, or displeasures and discomforts, not by their actual effects, but by suggestion.

There are certain classes of persons whose intellectual labours are characterised by suggestibility in a very marked degree, as, for example, authors. What can flatter an author more than to hear that his novel made men and women laugh or weep, or was effective in creating good morals or wicked conduct? And what is the object of the dramatist and actor but to suggest certain thoughts and feelings to the audience,

o

to make them think, laugh, or cry, at his will? The transformed emotion may be suppressed and is usually not lasting, but with a few, it is sometimes strong enough to prevent their enjoying their supper and sleep that night.

Even in business, suggestion plays an important rôle. The best salesman is he who can dispose of goods that the purchaser did not intend to buy, at least not at the price asked. The best buyer is he who can make a man sell his goods at a figure which he regrets as soon as they part. The art of advertising depends almost entirely on its power of suggestion. The daily repetition of a statement suggests that the assertion is a fact.

Suggestion influences not merely our mental states, but can affect the bodily functions. It is a fact of observation that pleasant, joyful, exalting emotions are accompanied by a feeling of well-being and capacity, by an increase in the vital functions and an invigoration of the whole organism; while, by certain depressive and distressing emotions, the contrary effect is produced and the nutrition of the body suffers. Everyone knows how the receipt of an unpleasant letter may make him lose all appetite for food and even cause him indigestion or headache, how fear may actually paralyse the muscles and keep him "rooted to the spot," how sudden shock will sometimes result in instant death, how long-continued grief or mental strain will sap the strength of the body. On the other hand, the mental disposition can be influenced by the bodily functions. Nobody is constantly the same self. We vary not only at different periods of our life, but on different days, according to our bodily state ; sometimes sanguine, sometimes gloomy ; sometimes genial, sometimes reserved ; sometimes apathetic, sometimes energetic. It is evident, therefore, that not only can the body be weakened through the agency of the mind, but it can be strengthened also by the same agency.

We are constantly influencing others and are constantly influenced by others ; but not only does mind act on mind, our mental states influence our bodily states and our bodily states influence our mental states. It is the scientific study of this action and reaction which has been taken up by numerous expert psychologists within recent years, and the results of which are being utilised nowadays by physicians in the treatment of disease under the name of *psychotherapy*.

The first essential for successful psychotherapy is that the patient have faith in the skill, the judgment, and the honesty of his medical adviser. If the patient lacks confidence in the physician he is not likely to carry out his instructions with that accuracy and exactness of detail which is at all times the secret of success. The physician, observing that the patient fails to obey him, loses his interest in the case, and unfortunately the patient is the sufferer under these circumstances. It is the patient who first acts psychically on the physician; and the manner in which the patient first acts towards the physician is quite as important a factor in successful psychic treatment as is the demeanour of the physician himself. Where there is no psychic contact the enthusiasm, the joy in one's work, diminishes. Hence it is this psychic contact which plays the determining rôle in psychotherapy. Without it medicines may be administered and surgical operations performed effectively; but successful suggestions cannot be implanted.

Wherever this psychic contact evolved from sympathy is present, it will not be difficult for the physician to extend that measure of tranquillity and patience which the nature of psychotherapy demands. This very demand, in fact, makes the practice of psychotherapeutics impossible for many physicians. Time and patience are factors of the greatest importance. To listen to the never-ending complaints of nervous patients is always a tax on both time and patience; but he who tries to hurry his patient, he who receives these complaints restlessly, without interest, or even with a hint that the complaints are foolish or imaginary, will never achieve the slightest success in this form of treatment. There are no fancied ills. There are physical ills and mental ills. Mental ills are just as real as physical ills. A person may be ailing because he persuades himself that he is ailing; but in that case his mind is so affecting his body that he is actually ailing physically, though the cause of the trouble is mental.

If the patient feels that he has not confidence in the doctor he has consulted, the best thing for him to do is to seek the advice of a physician in whom he has confidence, and to follow out his treatment, for one, two, or three months if need be, until the desired result is obtained. On the other hand, if he feels that he is losing rather than gaining ground, he would be foolish to continue any mode of treatment which is delusive, useless, and unsatisfactory.

This is of all things the most important. Many a patient becomes chronic, when he might have been cured long before, simply because of

the advice of his too anxious friends to consult
this man or that, or to take this or that quack
medicine, which cured Mr. So-and-so when everybody had given him up. I need scarcely say that
this is very unfortunate for the patient.

The difference between a successful doctor
and another who, perhaps with greater mental
gifts and larger knowledge, fails to win the
confidence of patients is mainly one of personality. The man who impresses sufferers and their
friends with belief in himself will—assuming him
to be honest—do far more good than he who,
whatever may be his scientific attainments, has
not the power of inspiring faith ; in a word, the
miracle of cure—in the class of cases with which
we are here dealing—is largely wrought by
psychotherapy, of which the most important
element is the personal influence of the physician,
by which he is able to soothe the patient's fears,
allay his anxieties, make him face the situation
calmly so that he may not use up any of his
vital force in useless worry, but, on the contrary,
employ all his available psychic energy in helping
nature to overcome whatever disturbance there
is within the organism.

The mental element in disease is a universal
and constant fact, but it prevails in different
cases to a different extent. I could relate

remarkable cases of cures by mental impressions only. There are no two cases alike; and not only are the easily recognisable differences of sex and age, occupation and education, financial means, temperament and capacity, decisive; but all the subtle variations of prejudices and beliefs, preferences and dislikes, family life and social surroundings, ambitions and prospects, memories and fancies, diet and habits must carefully be considered. Every element of a man's life-history, impressions of early childhood, his love and his successes, his diseases and his distresses, his acquaintances and his reading, his talent, his character, his sincerity, his energy, his intelligence—everything germane to the individual—ought to determine the details of the psychotherapeutic method. As it is impossible to determine all those factors by any sufficient enquiry, most of the adjustment of method must be left to the instinct of the physician, in which wide experience, solid knowledge, tact, and sympathy must be blended. Even the way in which the patient reacts on the method will often guide the instinct of the well-trained psychotherapist. The securing of personal information is of the utmost importance, because very often details of life and habits are discovered that can be so modified by instruction as to bring about a disappearance of unfavourable influences.

In the next place, let me emphasise the importance of a correct diagnosis in each case. It is as important to know what sort of a patient has a disease, as what sort of a disease a patient has. This does not mean merely determining the name of the disease ; it means obtaining a complete grasp of the patient's condition—why is he ill ; what prevents him from getting well ; what, if any, cause is still in operation ? Indeed, I am realising more and more that the successful psychotherapist must be first of all a skilled physician with a wide experience of men and women, not alone in disease, but also in health. Often some departure from proper ways of physical living will be found to be the starting-point. It may have been unavoidable when it occurred, or have been thought so at least, or more likely not thought about at all until the mischief was done.

Every case needs a special method and is in a way amenable to special procedures of verbal suggestion. All who have had practice among nerve patients know how much, in spite of very many points of resemblance, they really differ from one another in their tendencies, their sensitiveness, their character, their social aspirations, and their degree of intelligence; all of which are conditions that require from the physician, if he is to conduct the psychical treatment well, the most varied modes of address and manner. Consequently, before undertaking the psychical treatment of a nerve patient, we want to enquire not only into his history, his hereditary and personal antecedents, but also into the persons around him, the circumstances in which he first became ill and the real causes, moral or other, of his nervous exhaustion.

Analysis will often discover as the fundamental difficulty a sort of derangement of moral perspective. Trifles have come to occupy the foreground so completely that they obscure or altogether hide the larger and more important things beyond them. This is often because trifles do really and naturally occupy too large a share of his daily attention. The application of a little reasoning power to the consideration of such matters will, if the trouble be not too far advanced, reduce things to something like their proper perspective.

The mind and will of nervous patients is essentially weak and vacillating; hence arises the necessity for the controlling influence and guiding efforts of a will superior to their own.

What they want is disciplined treatment, under someone who, whilst having plenty of sympathy, can mix it with firmness and authority, so as to check the ramifications of disordered feeling and make the patient realise how to help himself. Where worry has played a prominent part in the causation of the patient's illness, and where it has been impossible to remove its source, the physician's task becomes a formidable one and will necessitate the exercise of the finest tact, founded upon a wide knowledge of human nature and of the various moral agencies which may be brought beneficially to bear upon it. It will do little good to tell this type of patient that he should not worry ; he knows as much himself, and, if he does not, his relatives or his friends have told him so long before he has reached the physician. They have also told him, in a spirit of genuine sympathy, that he should cease to think so much about himself, or that he ought to take a rest, or become interested in some hobby or in outdoor sports. Perhaps they have even lent him books, which he has read with hopeful diligence, about the value of optimism and of cheerfulness and self-control, with well-meaning hints as to the best method of culti-vating these estimable qualities. But in the end it has come to nothing, and why ? Because it is merely touching the fringe of the problem. What this man wants to know is, not that he should cease to worry, which is obvious, but *how* he is to cease to worry. And whoever can answer this problem gets at the root of the matter. Discouraged, weary, pessimistic, the patient comes to the psychotherapist asking, though he does not know it, for a practical philosophy of life. His own has broken down; or else he had never anything worth the name and never really felt the need of it until the present crisis brought him sharply to the realisation that such a thing is indispensable.

The patient has to be taught to think for himself and how to exercise MENTAL DISCIPLINE. As a rule he is complaining that he lacks decision, cannot concentrate at will, and that his thoughts are uncontrolled and wandering. Mental discipline gives force and efficiency to the mental powers, and strength to character. The patient is also likely to admit that he has got into a mental groove from which he cannot extricate himself. He is likely to admit that he has lost all interest in subjects that do not directly concern himself; but he may be unwilling to believe, or may even resent the suggestion, that his mental state is due to a large extent to his never having thought for himself and having taken all his thoughts second-hand, and thus having given his brain no work to do. That is how he became introspective and watched the internal working of his bodily machinery, to which the original and busy man pays little or no attention.

Of course, when the attention is fixed exclusively upon a diseased idea, it is very difficult for suggestion to find an entrance into the brain. Therefore the preliminary to all successful treatment is to remove unfavourable suggestions—mostly due to imperfect knowledge—before favourable suggestions are made. It will require considerable patience and perseverance to succeed ; but even with very obstinate patients there is a way of making an impression on the brain, and once an entrance is gained into the fortress of the mind, the gates for the admission of other impressions can be widened and widened till all resistance is broken.

The morbid ideas of the patient are the result of irritation of certain brain cells. It is not the idea itself, but the recurrence of the idea, which is morbid. Hence it is not always advisable to go direct against his ideas, but rather to try to direct the current of his thoughts into other channels. It is wonderful how sometimes a single impression made upon the mind by means of suggestion, a single hopeful idea introduced into it, may suddenly change the whole current of feeling and divert it from a morbid into a healthy channel. If we can once fix the attention upon any belief, or a happiness which is capable of attainment, we have made easy the way to recovery. If we can inspire by our assurance any glimmering hope of restoration, we have ministered powerfully to composure and serenity of mind and entered on the path that leads to ultimate cure.

In order to gain mental control, the cultivation of a hopeful spirit is of importance. Pessimism as a working principle of life is utterly bad from the point of view of mental stability. Human nature, as a general rule, absolutely needs for its continual mental health the support of an inspiring optimism. Those who look for trouble will always find it knocking at the door. I do not mean to convey, however, that all men have it in their power to be optimistic or pessimistic, just as they wish. That is not so. These conditions of feeling, to a large extent, come by temperament; but most men also have some choice in this as in other affairs of life. It is a wholesome determination not to allow the pinpricks of life to upset one.

The patient must be taught how to forget his troubles. We all try to remember too much.

We are cultivating the memory but not the art
of forgetfulness, which is equally important.
A well-trained memory is a very useful faculty
to possess, but if the health is sound and the
brain clear the impressions we receive will in
any case be more vivid and therefore more
lasting. A defective memory is often a sign of
disturbed health; and when this is attended to,
no artificial aids for improving the memory will
be necessary. The patients under consideration
too often remember what they should forget.
To let their disappointments, their failures, their
disagreeable experiences, linger in their minds,
not only dissipates their mental energy, but
reacts upon their body, impairing digestion,
disturbing sleep, and the general health suffers
in consequence. Forgetting is a splendid mental
calisthenic and a good medicine for these
patients. When the remembrance of unpleasant
happenings crowds into their mind, they should
use their will-power and turn their thoughts to
happier things. Let them take up a book and
read, or go out into the fresh air. Let them fill
the mind so full of other matters that there will
be no room for the disagreeable memories.
Let them go to sleep every night with the
thought of pleasant things before them and
begin the next day as though it was the first

day of their life and their only day, and let them make this day a record of sweet memories. To forget—that is what they need. Just to forget—themselves, their petty annoyances, their bitter disappointments, their mental difficulties, their bodily sensations. Let them learn to forget, make a study of it, let them practice it. Let them become experts in the art of forgetting what is not worth remembering, and they will add immeasurably to the health of both mind and body.

Not alone can functional disorders be benefited by suggestion, but various symptoms of organic disease can be also efficiently relieved. In all cases of serious organic disease there is a strong nervous element. The patient is apt to be agitated, perhaps he sleeps badly, or there may be pain. Now, if we can soothe the nervous system, secure sleep, and remove pain—and we can do all this—we are going a long way to improve the patient's condition. If we can alleviate the symptoms we have achieved a great deal. If, for instance, pain is disturbing digestion, rest, and the general mental capacity, the relief of pain places the patient on an altogether different footing from that on which he was before. In the same way with sleeplessness. If we can relieve sleeplessness in many cases the fundamental cause of that sleeplessness may be better treated. But as long as sleeplessness persists we are unable to attack the real cause. Often an illness is made worse by the fears of the patient. By suggestion treatment we can calm and quieten the patient's natural apprehension, and thus avert the worst effects of a disease.

Suggestion treatment does not constitute the entire psychotherapy. To apply it successfully we must use scientific methods of PSYCHO-ANALYSIS and synthesis, that is to say, we must dissect the mental tendencies of the patient until we find the real root of his trouble, and we must give them a new direction, together with moral therapy and hygienic physical measures. When we analyse the mind of the patient, it is often found that some painful experience in early life, of which he has lost recollection, has brought about a mental conflict and is still exercising an influence, though unconsciously, on his present thoughts, feelings, and actions, and is the source of his nervous derangement. In some cases the mere confession gives relief, and in others the fact that the hidden influence is brought under conscious mental control brings contentment, secures the proper mental adjustment, and leads to recovery.

Many physicians claim to use psychotherapy

who use only the method of PERSUASION, which consists of explaining to the patient the true reasons for his condition and making an appeal for the reform of his habits. This does very well in the simpler cases when done methodically, but it is my experience that by the time most nervous patients come to the physician, they have got beyond the influence of mere persuasion and require not only to be told to reform their habits, but to be shown *how* to reform them. Often they know perfectly well where they have offended, but lack the power to break themselves of their unhealthy physical or mental indulgences. We may correct errors of interpretation by persuasion, but to eradicate pathological convictions and to combat apprehensions, " suggestion " treatment must be employed.

In both methods, that of persuasion and that of suggestion, the mental mechanism, which has engendered the nervous disorder, must be taken apart bit by bit and be built up again on a rational basis by the process of RE-EDUCATION. We must show the patient in what way he has sinned ; how much his preoccupations, his reproaches, and remorses are exaggerated, and how useless they are ; what is the exact origin of his auto- and hetero-suggestions ; we must show him his errors of

P

interpretation of pathological phenomena, and what is the influence which emotional causes exert upon him. We must get the patient to realise his previous misconceptions, must uproot undesirable habits, which bad education, imitation, neglect, etc., have developed in him ; we must teach him to minimise his difficulties, to stop the magnification of trifles, and to gain self-control ; in short, we must aim at bringing about a rational mental adjustment.

It will be seen that it is not by any one method, but rather by a combination of the various methods which constitute psychotherapy, that we can hope to restore the patient to health. But what I wish to lay particular stress on is that in our successful teaching of self-control and mental discipline lies the future happiness of the patient and the prevention of his relapse.

CHAPTER XIV

THE METHOD OF APPLYING "SUGGESTION" TREATMENT

DIRECTIONS FOR AUTO-SUGGESTION

SUGGESTIBILITY is, as we have seen, a characteristic of all human beings, but there are methods which increase that suggestibility. Let me describe the one method which I have found almost invariably successful.

The patient is put in a comfortable position on a couch or arm-chair, in a quiet room, is asked to breathe regularly and deeply, and to compose himself in such a way as to bring about thorough relaxation of his muscles. The relaxation of the body and cessation from any voluntary muscular contraction is intended to stop the numerous leaks of nervous energy, and the regular deep breathing is to purify the blood and favour its circulation through the brain. All victims of despondency, all downcast and crestfallen people are shallow breathers.

The patient is then asked to gaze intently for

a while on some object, a picture, crystal, or subdued light, or to listen attentively to a monotonous sound, and to concentrate his thoughts thereon. This process helps to prevent the eyes from wandering all round the room and seeing the pictures, books, and furniture ; it helps to prevent other sounds being heard, shuts out distracting and exciting thoughts, prevents the mind from wandering, and produces a passive subjective condition suitable for suggestion and auto-suggestion. In very susceptible subjects a state of drowsiness may be produced, the eyelids may get heavy, when the patient will find it a relief to close his eyes and rest in a peaceful condition. In recent years this state of abstraction with relaxation has been spoken of as the hypnoidal state, because it is a state which resembles the preliminaries of sleep.

By the concentration of his attention we have put the subject in the condition of objective passiveness, in which the brain is at rest, the muscles are relaxed, all distracting thoughts are warded off, and the mind is completely absorbed to the exclusion of all external sensations. We have done the same as any man does in ordinary circumstances when he wants to concentrate on a subject ; he stops people talking to him and withdraws his attention from distracting sounds and all outside impressions for a while. An orator trying to make a speech to a roomful of talking people will not make very much impression ; but when his audience has been quieted, the ideas he presents will have some definite weight. In suggestive therapeutics the physician is the orator and the restive audience is represented by the turbulent thoughts of the patient.

We can now proceed to talk to the patient about his ailment, reassure him of his power to control his cravings, and to put away doubts and questionings which are irrational and entirely due to habitual tendencies that he has allowed to grow on him. All conceptions and ideas which we put forth are such as would appeal to the patient's reason, and do not come into collision with either his convictions or his feelings. For this purpose it is of course absolutely necessary to know what chords are likely to respond, and how we may build up the disintegrated personality. We explain to the patient the true reasons for his condition ; we show him in what way he has erred, what are the faults of his character and reasoning that brought about his present condition. We point out to the patient how much his preoccupations and reproaches and remorses are exaggerated, and how useless they are. We endeavour to establish confidence in himself, and to awaken the different elements of his personality which will enable him to regain self-control. We try to get the patient to turn his attention away from that which is painful and concentrate it upon what is agreeable and hopeful, to think of other and higher things than his own person, to control and order his thoughts and sensations that he may dominate them, and not be dominated by them. By the concentration of attention, the patient also forgets his internal sensations.

Just as pain can be made more acute by thinking of it, so it can be diminished by withdrawing the attention from the painful part. From the candidate in a competitive examination who forgets his toothache till he comes out of the examination room, to the soldier in action unconscious of the bullet wound till he faints from loss of blood, we have instances enough of intense concentration of attention on other events which has often made the resolute spirit altogether unconscious of conditions which would have been appalling to the ordinary man.

The patients do not lose consciousness ; they know what is taking place, though they may close their eyes and be willing to abstract their minds. The suggestion given is received by them in full consciousness; it does not escape from the control of their personality. And if they are docile subjects, convinced of the intellectual superiority of the physician, quite disposed in consequence to obey him, and vividly impressed by the method and by what they expect of it, it is easy to understand that they accept and carry out the " suggestion " that has been given to them. But this suggestion is, on ultimate analysis, only a suggestion received in the waking state, facilitated perhaps by the belief of the invalid in the efficacy of this mode of treatment and by the ceremonial associated with it. This form of treatment presents no dangers. The physician does not impose his will upon the patient; he acts only as a guide and teacher to enable him to discipline himself and to co-ordinate his scattered forces. It is certain that suggestion treatment, thus understood and applied, is able to render real service, as the examples quoted in the next chapter will show.

In this subconscious state any resolution that is passed by the subject is likely to be carried into action. Thus a person, whose will has become so defective that he is unable to break himself of a certain habit, can determine in that

state that he will no longer give way to it.
He states to himself the reasons why he ought
not to give way to it, why it would be positively
disastrous for him to go on as he has done—
and, indeed, that man will find, when the
temptation occurs again, that all his reflections are so vividly brought before him that
he will have no difficulty in resisting it.

We do not know why the resolutions made in
this state should have such a powerful effect;
we do not know, for the mechanism of the brain
machine is still a mystery to us. But that the
brain is capable of working unconsciously sometimes more efficiently than in the conscious state,
of that we have several examples. Thus it
happens sometimes that, when we try to recall
a name, we fail to remember it in spite of the
most determined efforts. We leave off thinking
about it and begin doing something else, and after
a few minutes the desired name is remembered,
as if of its own accord. The lesson we can draw
from this is that we should not be disappointed
if an effort of will fails, for the brain can act
intelligently without our being conscious of the
manner in which it works. The effort made
has been enough to set in motion our mental
activity in a manner unknown to us and to
make the missing word reappear in consciousness,

while our thoughts, at the actual time, seemed occupied with other subjects. Again, many persons can wake at any time they desire and find that, for this purpose, they need only fix their attention on the hour determined for a few moments before going to sleep. Similarly we can produce profound modification in ourselves by simply affirming what we desire. By keeping a particular thought vividly in our minds just at the moment of going to sleep, once sleep has supervened this idea will continue to develop and unfold itself without effort; and what is more, will often, thanks to the state of mental concentration, do so with more logical precision than would have been the case in the waking state.

Why is the time before going to sleep so well adapted for suggestion and auto-suggestion ? Because we are then in a dark and silent room, our eyes are shut to all visual impressions, the muscles are relaxed, and our body is in comfort, and we have dismissed all disturbing thoughts from our mind. This is exactly what is done in our treatment. The patient is installed where nothing can distract his senses or excite his mental faculties, his attention is completely released and therefore able to be directed to any idea upon which he is told or chooses to concentrate; and experience has taught us that under such conditions, the idea thus strengthened has its power of realisation greatly increased.

It is not absolutely necessary to wait until going to sleep for the exercise of auto-suggestion. After a little practice, we are able to concentrate for suggestion at any time and anywhere during the day by just isolating ourselves for a moment, and concentrating the mind on the suggestion. The willing should not be intense, there should not be any strain or struggling. It ought rather to be like a quiet, firm desire, impressed clearly and with conviction. The attention is focussed upon it, and then the idea is dismissed; and, although conscious attention is diverted from it, the idea realises itself unperceived.

As before mentioned, we are most susceptible to psychic suggestion at the moment when we are on the verge of sleep. A man who is ambitious for himself will take advantage of the opportunity this offers; and, when he goes to sleep, will make sure that the thoughts admitted into his mind are strong and healthy thoughts—thoughts of joy, of success, and accomplishment. This is not romance. It is certain fact that a man can make suggestions to himself at this time, and that there will be a positive effect for good upon the spirit and efficiency of his life. It will be seen that this state is very similar to the one a devout person is in when offering a prayer; and, like a genuine prayer, a genuine resolution for reform, in the subconscious state, strengthens the moral qualities and increases the nervous energy that helps the recovery from disease.

Now, in ordinary people, this power of suggestion does not come of itself; it must be educated. If this auto-suggestion were so easy, the patient would never have drifted so far as he has done. He requires the assistance of a physician, who has the right judgment of his psychic condition, his individual qualities, constitution, temper, disposition, and the mood he happens to be in at the time, and who must possess, of course, vast patience, abundant good nature, and tact. Some physicians fail in trying to use this treatment either because they are not trained for it, or they cannot judge the suitability and suggestibility of the patient for it, or give the proper suggestions in the right manner. Others again, when using psychotherapy, ignore the physical needs of the organism, which should be first attended to.

If the suggestionist is an expert, he will know how to *re-educate* his patient by introducing into the stream of mental life new and healthy complexes, sound ambitions, and hopeful visions of the future, which henceforth affect the whole personality. The physician, having previously searched the mind of the patient for the source of his disorder in the course of listening to his complete story, and having discovered the mental attitude of the patient toward his ailment and the false point of view which has resulted in the neurosis, now sets forth the right way to regain health and to effect a readjustment to life. As already insisted on, a necessary condition is a thorough understanding of the individual, his past life, his aims and desires, in a word, the contents of his inner world. In gaining this knowledge, we also learn his false conceptions of his own state, which themselves help to perpetuate his nervous state. One further step is to remove these by substituting for them correct ideas and by fixing them firmly in the mind. Finally, we must take up his special problems, his work, his domestic life, his pains and aches, his obsessive ideas, his special habits, in short, everything which enters into the orbit of his existence.

The patient is taught how to concentrate, how to focus on any given subject, and he is now counselled to do the same throughout the day : to focus his attention on whatever he has in hand, whether it be matters of business or pleasure. He is led to adopt new habits, to gain new interests and enthusiasms in harmony with his nature and possibilities, and to become absorbed in them. He is told also that, when he leaves the room, he is to use his powers of observation ; to notice on his way home and wherever he may go all objects that may interest him, to be on the look-out for them, so that he may have no opportunity for self-introspection, and may not be disturbed by any thoughts which are undesirable or un-welcome to him.

After the suggestions, resolutions, and auto-suggestions have been made, the patient is asked to dismiss the whole subject from his mind and to try to sleep naturally for a few minutes ; or, at all events, to remain in a condition of repose for a while before getting up.

This method has the advantage that nearly everybody can be subjected to it. It is different from that of hypnotism, since the person is not sent to sleep and no suggestions need necessarily be made by the operator, but by the patient himself in accordance with his own ideas, and he is increasing his own will-power. The usual objection to hypnotism was that it deprived a

person of his will. In the suggestion treatment
there need be no such apprehension, for its whole
efficacy lies in the operator strengthening the
will of the patient. For example, in many of the
disorders we have mentioned, we have a lack of
control over the powers which constitute mind
and character. By suggestion treatment we
restore that control, and teach the patient
mental discipline. Our treatment is therefore
educational. Re-education is the most important
of the therapeutic processes. Such a patient
has learned how to help himself, and he need
not fear a relapse to his old condition.

The ailments in which psychotherapy is of the
most conspicuous value are those characterised
by pain, insomnia, abnormal nervous irritability,
nervous tremors and spasms, depression of
spirits, phobias, obsessions, moral obliquity,
perversions of all kinds, drink and drug habits.

Individuality is not destroyed nor weakened,
but often greatly strengthened by the treatment.
A subject who has lost his evil habits, in whom
better ideals have been introduced, has lost
nothing of force of individuality; it has only
been improved and turned to better account.
Self-control has not been diminished, but, on
the contrary, the subject has been made able to
do the thing which in his best moments he de-

sired to do, but was not able to accomplish
unaided.

Patients who are addicted to perverse habits
which undermine their physical health and
destroy their mental energy are readily cured by
this method, the only condition is their willing
co-operation. Unfortunately a good many of
them do not want to be re-educated and to be
taught how to exercise self-control. What they
want is the performance of a miracle. They
know nothing of suggestion treatment; but they
have heard of hypnotism, and see in it a cure
which requires no personal effort. They would
like to rely on the doctor rather than on themselves. Many a patient addicted to alcohol,
drug-taking, or other bad habit has come to me
hoping that I would merely look at him to
send him to sleep and he would wake up in a
few minutes or half an hour completely cured.
True, such miracles have been performed; but
they are just rare enough to be miracles. Only
if the patient is willing to submit to the regular
process of treatment though it cost an effort on
his part, and only if he is perfectly sincere in his
desire, can he be cured.

If we can succeed in getting a patient into a
passive condition, we can give him suggestions
which attack the unnatural impressions of his

subconscious mind, we can teach him to look with disgust on his former violations of nature, and to find pleasure in natural and healthy modes of life. We try to improve his character by suggestions of self-restraint, which will remain operative whenever temptation occurs. He carries out the instructions which we have given him because they are in accord with his altered subconsciousness, and so he passes on to a new and happy life—not only relieved but cured of the habits which bred disease. Surely to turn the wavering, the despondent, the drug-seeking, into the buoyant, the energetic, the independent, to snatch from the gloomy toils of melancholy, or from the bondage of alcohol, men and women who have many years of life before them, and to render those years active and happy to the individual and of benefit to the community ; to do this, surely, is to perform a task of which any physician may well be proud, and which is worthy of more recognition than the physician generally receives.

In conclusion, let me repeat the directions for auto-suggestion :—

1. The patient must practise first of all to get his mind into a state of peacefulness and calmness. Let him seek a quiet room where he is undisturbed, and let him take up a position

of ease, or lie comfortably on a couch, with all the muscles relaxed. Then let him breathe deeply and regularly, but without an effort. If thoughts run through his brain he is not to try to resist or control them, but just to give way to them. He is not to worry about them, but to surrender himself to them, as if he did not care. Resistance only increases the nervous tension. Non-resistance will soon put him at ease.

2. Having succeeded so far, the next time he is in that state of calmness let him try to think of something pleasant, something that delights him to contemplate, allowing his imagination free play. In this manner, he will gradually acquire the power of focussing on an idea, and of ignoring his external surroundings and internal sensations.

3. After being able to produce this condition successfully, he may in this state of calmness focus on something he wishes to achieve ; for example, to be able to sleep, to have freedom from bodily pain and discomfort, to become self-possessed or cheerful, or to be able to work hard without feeling weary, and to subdue irritability and the habit of worrying. He must be serious with his suggestion. His conviction must be in it, but there should be no strain, no tension, no struggling. It ought rather to be

Q

like a quiet, firm desire. Having expressed his
desire or resolution deliberately, he must dismiss
the subject and turn his thoughts again to his
work or whatever he has in hand, or simply rest
peacefully for a few minutes.

For example, in order to obtain sleep let the
patient get first of all into a condition of repose,
as already described, without tension of either
muscles or mind, and with no conscious effort;
then let him concentrate on the idea of sleep,
repeating to himself: "I shall sleep within a
few minutes soundly and uninterruptedly, and
undisturbed by any discomfort or pain, and I
shall wake at eight o'clock in the morning feeling
perfectly refreshed and cheerful." Having made
his suggestion with confidence in its success, let
him think no more about it, but remain perfectly at ease; and if sleep does not come at
once he must not be disappointed, but should
think of something pleasant, allowing his imagination free play. If *positive* thoughts, such as
"I shall sleep," prove unsuccessful, let him try
negative thoughts, such as : "I shall not be able
to keep awake." He may think of something
else then, or try to read a book; and he will soon
find that he is getting drowsy and will fall
asleep.

CHAPTER XV

EXAMPLES OF "SUGGESTION" TREATMENT

THE difficulties the psychotherapist has to contend with are many. The first and most important condition for his success is that the patient has faith in him. But how is this possible when the patients are sent to him—not infrequently—only after all other methods have failed, and their belief in doctors in general has been considerably shaken and their resources have been strained ? The psychotherapist is then expected—by some, at all events—to succeed at a single interview ; and if he fails, the whole method of psychotherapy is condemned.

There is much ignorance, too, as to the kind of cases that would be benefited by such treatment; and the mistake is frequently made, more by patients than by doctors, of regarding the various methods of psychotherapy as an exclusive system of treating functional disease, as if it were the sovereign remedy for all nervous

227

disorders. I do not suggest that every case of nervous disorder should receive this form of treatment, nor do I wish it to appear that every case treated by suggestion is always cured. But considering the supposed wonders of the various cults of faith healing, I want to show that psychical treatment can be carried out by a qualified physician in a legitimate and scientific manner with absolute success and freedom from danger.

Another obstacle is that we are sometimes forbidden to give any medicine, or use any other measure whatsoever, to improve the constitution of the patient. Yet it must be obvious, that, while the patient is in an exhausted state and his nerves are irritable and react too quickly, we cannot secure that placidity of mind which is so necessary for our treatment. Medical psychotherapists, unlike other mental healers, do not rely on psychical influence alone, but employ other measures as well; for even where it is simply a question of curing a patient's " bad habits," his physique is likely to have suffered, and we have to restore not merely the mental condition, but the health of the organisation with which mind is connected and upon the normal state of which its soundness depends. It is the duty of the physician, when called upon to treat a patient, to carry out not one, but all of the measures which have been shown by years of experience to be advantageous. Medicinal, hygienic, dietetic, physical and moral measures, have all to be employed according to the individuality of the patient and the nature of his complaint. We must not, as Christian Scientists and other cults do, relegate tried methods to the dust-heap, but recognise that, even if there be no actual disease of the body, the patient, owing to his habitual indulgence of morbid thoughts or habits, has weakened his constitution, and may suffer from a state of nervous exhaustion or irritability, which require treatment on established lines. Psychical treatment alone, and physical measures alone, are insufficient; the two must be combined, and for the proper application of both, medical as well as psychological knowledge is essential. The patient who has been treated by psychotherapy alone is likely to have a relapse, because the constitutional condition which has given rise to the complaint has not been attended to. The patient who has received constitutional treatment only, whether by medicine or any other physical measure, may still be subject to his morbid thoughts, because no attempt has been made to cure him of his unhealthy mental habits.

The following are examples of the treatment
of nervous disorders by psychotherapy :—

Case of *Nervous Exhaustion with Imperative
Ideas and Loss of Will-Power* :—

Successful merchant, aged thirty-six, of splendid
physique, explained that he was afraid of going
to a theatre or any public hall for fear that he
would shout " Fire," and that he had to force
his handkerchief in his mouth to prevent himself
from doing so. At the same time, he suffered
from complete indecision, could not make up
his mind to do anything ; and if it was made up
for him, he was sure to stop in the middle of any
action he commenced. For example, his business
necessitated his travelling from London to
Glasgow, and he delayed for days before he
could make up his mind to do so, and ultimately,
when he did start, he got out at Carlisle to return
home. Letters which had been written after
many efforts were repeatedly destroyed, and
finally, if they were fortunate enough to reach
the letter-box, he was anxious to reclaim them
from the post. Education of the will by means
of suggestion, assisted by some physical measures
to influence the source of his affection, restored
the patient in a few weeks.

Case of *Nervous Exhaustion with Insomnia :—*
Patient, a professional man, forty-eight years
of age, had to do unusual hard work and to
undergo considerable anxiety. The first symptom which he noticed was sleeplessness, which
gradually got worse. He either did not go to
sleep at all on getting into bed, or, if he dropped
asleep from utter weariness, he woke up again
in about half an hour and lay restless during
the remainder of the night. Besides this, he
complained of a feeling of great exhaustion, total
disinclination to work, and to bodily exercise
of any kind, of weakness in the back and pain at
the nape of the neck. He was easily excited and
worried by little things, and extremely intolerant
of noise or of being asked any questions. He
was often troubled with a sense of vague alarm
and distressing sensations in the head. He
disliked his meals and generally suffered from
flatulence. The patient was treated with the
application of the constant current to the spine
and head, and psychotherapeutic influences were
brought to bear during the treatment. He almost
immediately began to sleep well; and after two
weeks the patient felt like another man, being
able to exert himself both mentally and bodily,
to enjoy his meals, and to take an interest in the
concerns of daily life,

Case of *Nervous Exhaustion with Headache, Giddiness, and Impaired Memory :—*

A lawyer, aged thirty-eight, had experienced considerable domestic anxiety, to which he attributed his illness. He complained of a sensation of weight and pressure at the top of the head and in the temples, and of giddiness. He felt a swimming sensation and "unsteadiness" in the head, especially on assuming the erect posture, which caused him sometimes to be uncertain and swaying in his walk. His memory and power of application were very much impaired. He was irritable to slight noises, easily excited, and on examination his reflexes were found exaggerated. Galvanism was applied to the spine and head with satisfactory results. The mental symptoms gradually yielded to "suggestion," and three weeks after the commencement of the treatment the patient was able to resume his work in excellent health.

Case of *Nervous Exhaustion with Lack of Concentration, Application, and Loss of Memory :—*

Patient, a captain in the army, aged thirty-three, was ordered home on leave from his Indian station, being unfit for work. Could not remember any orders, nor solve the simplest problem of tactics. " His mind was a blank," and " he felt weak all over," he said. Although he had already had ten months' rest, and was treated during that time, he had made no improvement. His last doctor sent him to me for treatment by suggestion. After ten days' treatment, patient was able to start work with a military coach, and in a month's time he left perfectly cured.

Case of *Agoraphobia* :—

A man, thirty years of age, found himself mixed up in an affair which gave him a great fright. Thereafter, although he had preserved his perfect lucidity of mind and directed his business as well as ever, he could not remain alone, either in the street or in a room and needed to be accompanied everywhere. If he did go out alone, which very rarely occurred, he found himself seized with a sense of anguish at the sight of a public square or of an open space of any considerable extent. If he had to cross one of the squares, he had the feeling that the distance was one of several miles and that he would never be able to reach the other side. This emotion diminished or disappeared if he went around the square following the houses, or if he was accompanied. A medicinal sedative and regular suggestion treatment put him right in a few weeks, and there was no recurrence of his complaint.

Case of *Chronic Headache :—*

Patient, forty-five years old, had repeated attacks of headache, one or two per week, during which he grew pale, and after a few minutes of agonising pain, in which he distorted his face and rolled his eyes, he appeared almost unconscious. He then revived, shaking all over. At the first two sittings, only sleep was suggested. On the third day, being fairly somnolent, a mild galvanic current was applied to the head, while explanatory suggestions were made as to the beneficial effect of electricity. On the fifth day, patient acknowledged the soothing effect of the current and went to sleep after the operation. On the seventh day he had completely recovered, and there was no return of his complaint, as shown by a report a month later.

Case of *Hypersensibility :—*

Gentleman, thirty-five years of age, after various financial and family troubles, had a nervous breakdown, and was treated by different physicians for a considerable period, and although better, was left with hypersensibility of nerves. The closing of doors in his house, the twittering of birds in his garden, the jarring of glasses carried on a tray, the dropping of even a light article, creaking boots, etc., all noises, however slight, whether real or anticipated, caused him intense agony and awful irritability. Patient submitted to treatment by suggestion. He retained full consciousness during my presence, but fell asleep afterwards, at first for a few minutes, then for a quarter, half, and a whole hour, waking up calm and composed. He noticed noises less and less, and after a fortnight he was able to resume his former occupations and pursuits.

Case of *Noises in the Head and Hearing of Voices* :—

Patient, a major in the army, forty years of age, suffered from insomnia, buzzing in the left ear, and the hearing of voices, which tortured him so much that he was afraid of going mad. No hereditary disposition nor previous illness. On examination it was found the power of hearing was not diminished and was equal on both sides. His ears had been previously examined by an aurist, who could discover no disease. At first he heard voices, conveying words of insult, at night only, thus preventing his sleeping. He suspected a neighbour of this and challenged him, but that gentleman proved that on those nights he had been away from home. Then he suspected others and got equally satisfactory explanations. He then recognised that these voices must be hallucinations ; but they became more and more distinct, and he began to hear them during the day and in the street. Then arose impulses to attack strangers, which he controlled only with difficulty. The voices always conveyed the same insults, quite close to him, and they were most distinct when he stopped his right ear up. Patient was convinced that he was suffering from hallucinations of hearing, yet he was full of anxiety lest he might give way to homicidal impulse. He was put in a state of somnolence, and suggestions were made to give him greater control over himself, minimising the significance of the hallucinations and lessening the distinctness of the voices. At the same time a mild galvanic current was applied to the left ear. This process was repeated for four weeks. All hallucinations had disappeared by then and the patient was able to resume his duties.

Case of *Nervous Exhaustion with Impotence* :—

Patient, aged forty-eight, journalist by profession, married for about a year, in consequence of overwork and anxiety got into a state of complete nervous derangement. He was utterly incapable of any mental or bodily exertion and had lost all virile power, which distressed him greatly. Horrible thoughts came into his head which rendered his life perfectly intolerable. His judgment and intellect were not impaired, but he had not the slightest control over the dreadful ideas which constantly flitted across his brain and made work absolutely impossible. One day he attempted suicide, but was saved by his wife, who brought him to me. I used suggestion treatment during the first week, and made the patient understand that there was nothing to worry about, that his want of virile power was entirely due to his nervous exhaustion and would return when his nervous system improved. The second week I applied galvanism to the spine daily, not neglecting at the same time to teach the patient the importance of mental discipline and the value of concentration. At the end of the second week patient had lost all his disagreeable thoughts, was cheerful in conversation, and at the end of the third week he returned to work feeling perfectly fit.

Case of *Nervous Exhaustion complicated by Dyspepsia* :—

Patient, a merchant, forty years of age, as a

result of overwork and anxiety had developed a neurasthenic condition, become somewhat hypochondriacal, and complained of severe dyspepsia. He consulted various specialists for gastric disorders, and their examination of the gastric juice, lavage of the stomach, and regulations as to diet had impressed still more strongly upon the mind of the patient the idea of a true stomachic affection. When I examined the patient, I certainly found distension due to flatulence; but the indigestion was mental in origin, and due in great measure to the fanciful diet the patient had indulged in since the commencement of his illness, and to his peculiar notions and antipathies. I ordered galvanic treatment to the stomach and, at the same time, began to influence his prejudices. The treatment was by no means easy; but after a few visits, the patient's common sense gained the upper hand, and from that time he made a rapid recovery.

Case of *Loss of Power and Shooting Pains in Legs* after motor-car accident :—

Patient, aged thirty-three, of nervous disposition, was in a motor-car accident two years before, from which he escaped with a shaking. He complained of a loss of power in his legs, and after a few days of severe shooting pains, he consulted a physician, who declared his affection to be of a functional nature. After taking some medicines and not getting better, he was recommended to try psychotherapeutics. I proposed combining galvanic treatment to the spine and lower limbs with " suggestion " treatment. He soon got better, gained power, and lost the painful sensations.

Case of *Functional Paralysis of Left Arm :*—

Talented young man, twenty-three years of age, after strenuous work at teaching and some early worry over his personal prospects, felt a sudden loss of power and sensation in his left arm and left leg. The lower limb recovered, but the arm remained powerless by his side. When lifted to the shoulder, it dropped heavily to the side. Sensation had returned. The doctor to the college and a specialist diagnosed functional paralysis; but no improvement resulting from their treatment, they recommended " suggestion " to be used. Success was achieved at the fourth sitting. The patient was then able to lift his left arm and to resist any attempts to pull it to his side. He preserved absolute control over his limb afterwards.

Case of *Stammering* :—

Solicitor, aged thirty-five, consulted me for general nervousness, self-consciousness, and stammering, which did not affect him always, but chiefly in the presence of clients, and actually interfered very much with his professional success. " I believe," he said, " that if I could only be relieved of the consciousness that I had ever stammered, I should stammer no longer." Patient had to attend a board-meeting of directors of a company that afternoon; so I used suggestion at once that he would not trouble at all about the events this afternoon, would forget that he ever was nervous and self-conscious, that he would now be self-reliant, and would speak on this occasion without any involuntary break in his voice and without any hesitation whatever. Patient was not quite so successful, but he acknowledged he got over the ordeal much better than he would have done if he had not come to me. Suggestions were then continued and his general nervousness was attended to; with the result that he got over his speech defect completely.

Case of *Hystero-Epilepsy* :—

Patient, a clerk, eighteen years old, had the first attack when ten years old, and the attacks had recurred about twice a week since. It was believed that he lost consciousness in these attacks, in which he fell to the ground, made irregular movements with his arms and legs and twitched his face ; it was noticed, however, he had never bitten his tongue nor injured himself in any way, nor did he sleep after the attack, as is the rule with genuine epileptics. He had been better for some two years, but relapsed six months later after a fright. My own observation : " Patient previous to attack gets very irritable, breathes heavily, gets into ' dreamy states,' talks indistinctly, falls with his eyes wide open, with twitching of his limbs and face; and after five minutes he appears exhausted, breathes again more quickly, and gets up in another two minutes as from a dream, wondering what has happened." I tried hypnotism in this case and succeeded immediately. At the first three sittings, patient was allowed to remain in deep sleep for an hour, without any suggestions being made, except that he, on waking up, would feel well and strong. On the fourth day, he was told a minute after the commencement of the sleep that he would wake up, open his eyes, know his surroundings, but would remain under my influence. He was questioned then about his attacks, and impressed with the desire to

R

control his premonitory symptoms of compression of the chest and irritability. He was shown how to breathe deeply, make his limbs rigid, including the arms and fingers, to put his feet firmly on the ground, and to " determine " not to have an attack. After some tests that he was really still under control, he was told to forget that it was I who had given him these instructions, but that he himself, when premonitory signs appeared, would get into these attitudes as if they originated with him, and feel quite determined and confident that he would defeat the attack. The sittings were continued for a fortnight on alternate days and then one a week for a month. Patient had no more attacks, and the premonitory symptoms occurred only twice during the first week and once the succeeding week ; after that they ceased. He reported himself as having kept well two years later.

Case of *Mental Torpor, Fugitive Pains, and Palpitation* from excessive cigarette smoking :—

Young man, aged twenty-eight, who became conscious of the injurious effect cigarette smoking had on him, and who had persistently tried to break off the habit, but failed, came to seek my aid. He told me he smoked incessantly from early morning till night, and that he could not

do his work as well as formerly, being disturbed
by pains and palpitation and a confused head.
I got him into a somnolent state, in which I told
him that he would control his inclination, that
he would reduce the number of cigarettes he
smoked to ten that day, and that he would wake
up with a feeling of encouragement and determination that this time he would succeed in
breaking his habit. On the following visit I
reduced the number to five cigarettes, and explained to the patient that the reduction would
already have the effect of clearing his head,
getting the heart more regular, and restoring
his health in general. By the end of the week
he had left off smoking altogether, and he reported some weeks after that he had not felt
the slightest inclination to smoke any more.

Case of *Drink Habit* :—

A curate, thirty-two years of age, suffering
from exhaustion and insomnia owing to prolonged overwork, took to secret drinking, but
was after a time found out and lost his position.
This blow weakened his self-control still more,
when his relatives interested themselves, and
after trying various homes for him brought him
to me for " suggestion " treatment. I ordered
a companion for him at once, prescribed a

medicinal sedative, and stopped all alcohol. Then I tried to induce the hypnotic state, but though I got no further than mere somnolence, I reasoned with him, explained to him that he would feel no ill-effects from having abstained, that he would feel perfectly content all day and sleep well at night, and that this improved condition without drinks would have the effect of convincing him that he could do without them, and would make him resolve earnestly never to touch alcohol again, not even under the pressure of unhappiness. The suggestions were repeated daily at first and then at prolonged intervals. Gradually he was allowed money of his own and to go out without his companion. After two months, the companion was discharged. The patient, who went to reside with a sister of his, still reported himself every few weeks for about a year. Then I used my influence with a clerical friend who takes a great interest in the reform of inebriates to give him another chance, and I have recently heard that he is doing well at his work and has had no relapse.

Case of *Morphio-Mania* :—

In this case morphia injections were ordered for severe pains in the leg after an accident in South Africa, and the doctor allowed the patient to go on with them when he wanted to return to England. Patient gradually got addicted to morphia, was in agony or at least could do no work without it. The plan on which I practised suggestion in this case was as follows : I ascertained that the strongest character-trait of the patient was his strong love for his son. By presenting to him a mental picture of his own degradation before his son, and the disgust the boy must feel at the sight of his depraved father, and by impressing him with the possibility of his premature death, and thus of not being able to direct the education of his son, nor see him grow up, and by other similar suggestions, the patient's reason and will-power grew strong enough to enable him to cease his pernicious habit, and it has not recurred again.

INDEX

WILLIAM BRENDON AND SON, LTD., PRINTERS
PLYMOUTH, ENGLAND